SHINE BRIGHTER EVERY DAY

Nourish Your Body, Feed Your Spirit, Balance Your Life.

Danah Mor

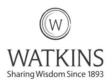

WATKINS
Sharing Wisdom Since 1893

YOU CANNOT PUT MORE DAYS IN YOUR LIFE, BUT YOU CAN PUT MORE LIFE IN YOUR DAYS.

This book is dedicated to you, who have the right to know the truth about what you are being sold and told, for your own vitality and quality of life. You have the right to choose a path, rather than walking one someone else created.
You have the right to shine bright.

Shine Brighter Every Day
Danah Mor

First published in the UK and USA in 2020 by Nourish, an imprint of Watkins Media Limited
Unit 11, Shepperton House,
83–93 Shepperton Road
London N1 3DF

enquiries@nourishbooks.com

Typeset in Futura, Cera Pro and Turbinado Pro
Colour reproduction by XY Digital
Printed in China

Commissioning Editor: Jo Lal
Managing Editor: Daniel Hurst
Editor: Sophie Elletson
Managing Designer: Francesca Corsini
Production: Uzma Taj
Commissioned artwork: Maya Mor and
   Pedro Salvador Mendes
Commissioned photography: Matt + Lena
   Photography

A CIP record for this book is available from the British Library

ISBN: 978-1-84899-380-8

10 9 8 7 6 5 4 3 2 1

Publisher's note: The information in this book is not intended as a substitute for professional medical advice and treatment. If you are pregnant or breastfeeding or have any special dietary requirements or medical conditions, it is recommended that you consult a medical professional before following any of the information or recipes contained in this book. Watkins Media Limited, or any other persons who have been involved in working on this publication, cannot accept responsibility for any errors or omissions, inadvertent or not, that may be found in the recipes or text, nor for any problems that may arise as a result of preparing one of these recipes or following the advice contained in this work.

nourishbooks.com

CONTENTS

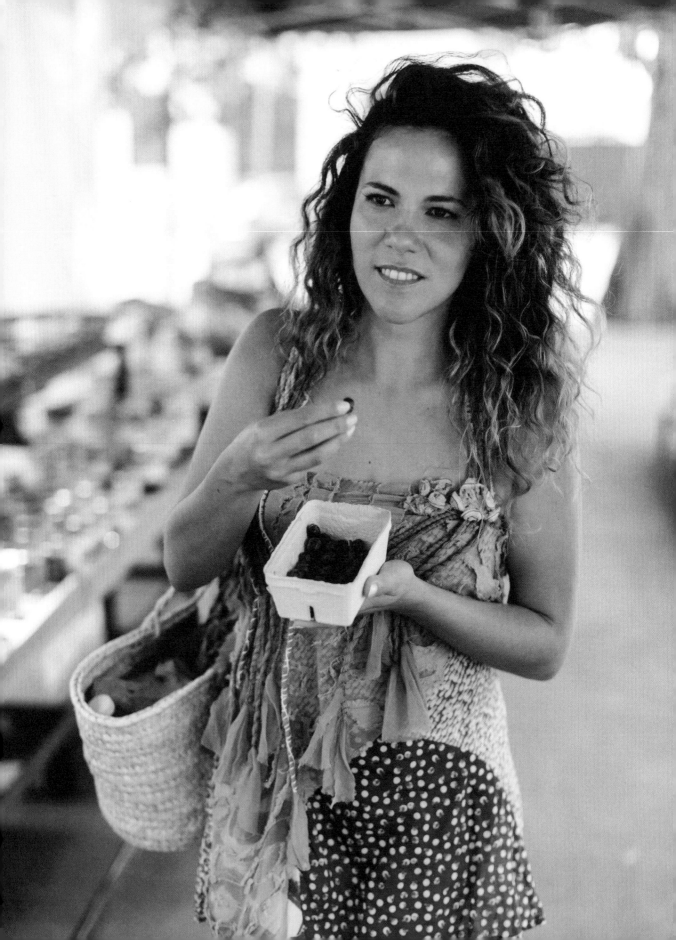

INTRODUCTION

If we knew how amazing our bodies were designed to feel, we wouldn't think twice about our choices.

How do you explain to someone driving a car from 1970 that the ride doesn't have to be uncomfortable, smell like petrol, or constantly break down? It's likely they're just happy their car gets them around. And even if it doesn't cost much to get it fixed, they will take some persuading to change to a newer model!

Most of us have become accustomed to disease, pain and discomfort in our bodies and minds. **We are happy enough to have a body that simply gets us around,** rather than making an effort to see how we could improve things for ourselves. Sometimes, even, we don't want to leave our comfort zone of discomfort and disease; we prefer not to know and just stick with the disease.

This book is about improving your quality of life, preventing disease, and manifesting the best version of yourself. It unlocks a lifestyle, a way of thinking – a state of being – that is in tune with your body, inspired by the unwritten laws of nature, cutting-edge modern nutrition science, the ancient wisdom of Ayurvedic medicine and my own personal experience.

I'm urging you to have the courage to be interested and try a few little steps to see how your body responds and thanks you.

You can only feel as good as you think you can.

When I was around thirteen, I lost a large portion of my vision, and this has given me a new perspective on life. Ultimately, it has shown me how many things are possible. Life is what you make of it. It's not what you have – it's what you make of what you have. I can't change my condition. But by perceiving my condition in a different way, I was able to overcome bigger barriers than most of us can imagine and as a result build a life that I love living. I did this by not focusing on my problem and what I couldn't see, but rather focusing on what I could see. And I realized that I actually see much more than many people. I realized just because we have ears, it doesn't mean we listen, and just because we have eyesight, it doesn't mean we look. The curiosity to look without projecting an illusion is harder than I ever imagined. Looking without expectation, with courage to see the truth, is one of the hardest things I have come to learn. Your willingness is your biggest asset; wanting to be or do anything is the beginning of truly becoming the driver of your own life.

VITALITY IS OUR BIRTHRIGHT

When it comes to our health, there is a lot of confusion and conflicting advice. What is vitality? What does it mean to be healthy?

How would you like to have the strength, courage and the capacity to mentally and physically live life to its fullest potential? What does this mean to you? Most of us don't really connect to what vitality really means to us on a physical and mental level.

Here are some ideas: to travel and live with ease, with no allergies, no stomach pains, no skin issues. To go swimming in the sea, go skiing or out dancing – always feeling strong and secure in body and mind. To run your business with energy and passion, to think without brain fog. To be able to run around with your children, nephews or grandchildren without pain or fatigue! To have strong, shiny hair, smooth, glowing skin and a resilient body. To feel confident from the inside out, at home in your own body. To feel satisfied and at peace with your life and your achievements. These are all signs of health and vitality.

Without health and vitality we start to lose out on life.

Believe it or not, vitality is our natural state. But I doubt many of us wake up and spring out of bed ready to seize the day! What has happened?

NATURE IS PERFECT

Nature is perfect by design and works in perfect balance. We are surrounded by everything we need. Water is filtered through the clouds and mineralized in the ground. Seeds are spread by the wind and feathers, sprouted by the rain to provide food for our consumption. Clean water, fresh air, nutritious delicious food and sunshine – we have it all; and then we have intuition and instinct that help guide us.

We live in an era where the main drive is profit. Unfortunately, this has changed the world for all of us. The choices that governments make regarding health, food regulations and safety are not for the good of our health, but the profit and success of business. This means that we can no longer trust the foods or other products on our supermarket shelves.

With the industrialization of our society and our modern-day consumer programming, we live from the outside in; we create external goals and expect to feel different. Here, our goal is to shine from the inside out, and reconnect with ourselves and with nature – because that is where we come from and only by truly understanding that connection can we really feel amazing and thrive again.

Many adults and children nowadays don't know where their food comes from. Most of us have never seen the vegetables we eat growing in the ground or on a tree – and many of us would be unable to recognize them in nature. The gap between us and nature needs to stop and reverse. We need to reconnect to nature – to our origin – if we want any chance of true health and vitality.

Of course, we're not talking about going back to the jungle (although it would be fun for a couple days!). But we do need to understand that the current models we live in are not set up in favour of people feeling content from the inside.

Our lives are limited by us and can equally be unlimited.

If we're given the conditions and tools to truly express our essence without limitations, restrictions or expectations, we may surprise even ourselves.

If you plant a tree in a junkyard in the middle of a polluted city, it may live forty years. Planted in the countryside, its lifespan could increase to three hundred years, and if planted on the windswept ridges of the Alps, or its perfect conditions, it may survive over two thousand years.

When a tree is given the optimal tools and environment to grow and express itself, the quality and span of its life improves drastically. Similarly, we can create the best conditions for ourselves. Neglecting the importance of these conditions, our life will be limited by ourselves; the only one that can create the conditions is you.

Most of us think we have little or no power to create change, but we do.

This book will show you how to create change, to make better, smarter, more fun choices.

Being interested and caring for your body, mind, and spirit may be the coolest thing you ever do!

MY INSPIRATION

From early on, it became clear to me that if I wanted anything in life, I had to work for it. My family were my inspiration in this. When they were young, my parents moved to a new country and built everything from the ground up – it had been my dad's dream to have a restaurant serving delicious, healthy, not-so-fast food, and they did it. Both my parents come from families that made the choice to move and change, to choose life over surrendering to death. My grandparents survived the holocaust by running away and saving their own lives – while their siblings didn't. My family have always shown me that nothing in life was impossible as long as you have the will and work hard to make it happen.

When people ask me where I'm from, I'm not sure how to answer. As a teen I struggled with my own identity, as I was from so many places. Mum is from South Africa, Dad is from Israel, I was born in Amsterdam and grew up in Portugal. I also spoke fluent English, Portuguese, Spanish and French. Today I speak seven languages. What I am sure of is that wherever I am in nature, I feel at home.

PASSION FOR FOOD

At home, if there was any abundance, it was with food! The fridge was always full and the house was flooded with delicious aromas. My family was known for our food – always fresh and nutritious! Both my parents' cultures revolve around food and hospitality. In mum's culture, meals are shared on a single platter in the centre of the table, with everyone leaning over to dig in – often without cutlery. Meals are about communing and sharing with friends and family. They are what keeps us together. Every event at home involves food and everyone loves to cook. My brother even became a Cordon Bleu gourmet Chef!

It was my mum who taught me about the relationship between food and the body, and how to listen to my body. As a kid, when my tummy ached, Mum always asked me, "What did you eat?" When I had a headache, Mum asked me if I had drunk enough water. I was constantly being shown that what I ate and drank were directly connected to how I felt. This made perfect sense to me even at an early age.

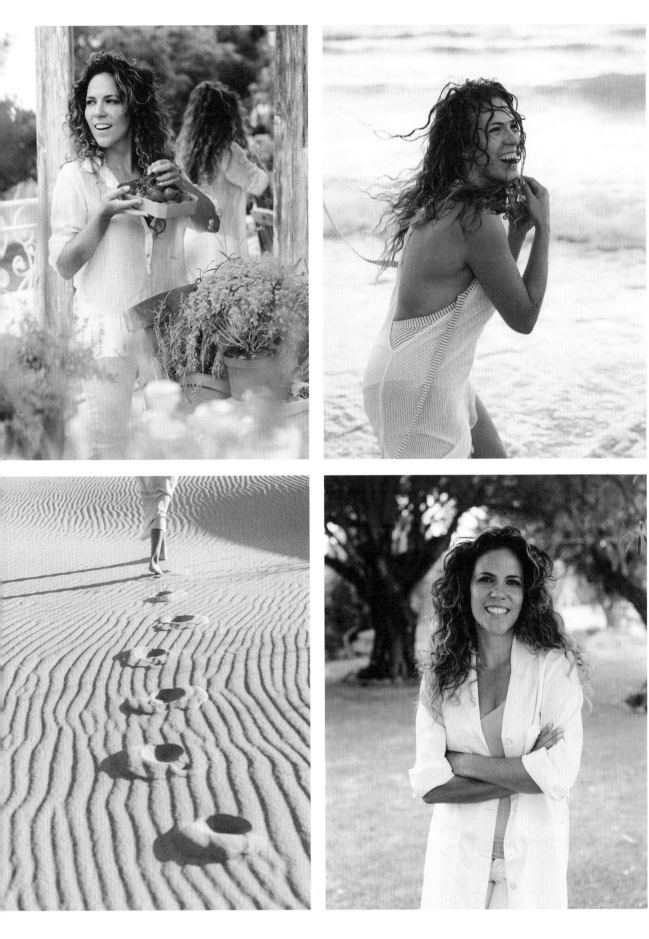

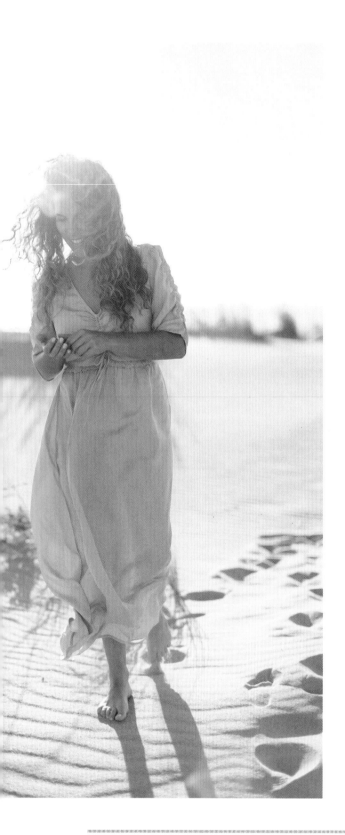

TRAVELLING TO FIND MYSELF

I have always loved to travel and, from my early teens, I would work in my parents' restaurant in the evenings and at weekends to save for my next adventure. For me, travelling is about discovering new ways of living and experiencing the world, and I have always loved immersing myself fully in new cultures. When my siblings and I were children, my parents would take us on wonderfully back-to-basics trips whenever possible – no five-star hotels for us! Travelling in this way meant that we would find ourselves fully immersed in indigenous cultures and natural ways of life. One of my most treasured memories is drinking and eating at an oasis in the middle of the Sinai desert with local Bedouins after riding camels and hiking through the desert. The food was so colourful – so many vegetables with such amazing flavours. Another of my most memorable voyages was to Yucatan, Mexico, where we spent time with native Mayans. I observed their natural ways of life and noticed where modern commodities interfered with their natural lifestyle; realizing this first hand made me aware that our modern world may be creating a gap between us and our natural source of vitality.

I feel so grateful and privileged to have had these experiences. Experiences that, to this day, continue to change the way I look and feel about food, society, happiness and life. As my perspective evolves, I understand that the true essence of anything is within each of us. I listen to stories of my parents, and their parents, making such courageous steps towards life, running from war, leaving their family behind. My grandpa fled during the night and jumped on a small fishing boat to cross the river. He had taught himself how to swim as a boy, so when the boat capsized he was able to swim to the other side. Stories like this make me realize just how much more comfortable my life is today. Sometimes we need less, not more – we need to simplify our perspective and reconnect to what our true soul desires, rather than being seduced and confused by the external world. All of us have the tools to re-build a life we love. My goal is to awaken your true essence and motivate you to express yourself, your true self (which you may not know yet).

Life is much simpler than we make it. At the end of the day, it's how you feel inside that creates a feeling of home; not what's on the outside. As you already know, when I was around thirteen, I lost a large portion of my eyesight. This was incredibly hard for me, but has also given me a new perspective on life. Ultimately, it has shown me how many things are possible. Everything is relative to how you think, and the only way to feel better is to open your mind and stop being conditioned by your thoughts. I realized this early on, when my eyesight started to disappear. It was as if I had to open my inner eyes and look deep within myself. I had to find courage, confidence and trust, even though I had little to hold on to on the outside. I couldn't see what I was used to seeing. I was losing my vision and it was scary. When you look within, you begin a new kind of conversation with yourself. When you look and listen inside, you create in-sight. Creating this stronger connection with myself was a foundation of what I call "feeling at home". When you feel at home inside of yourself, anywhere you place yourself can be home, because you are already home.

AYURVEDA, THE SCIENCE OF LIFE

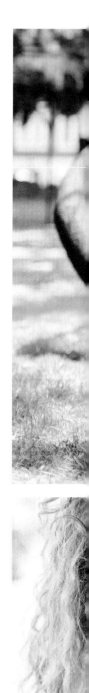

It was midday in mid-July and the sun was scorching hot over a Tel Aviv beach. Small heat rashes had broken out all over my body, and I was becoming irritable and moody.

I was nine years old when Mum introduced us to her dear friend, Dr Verma. We called him Verma G, the "G" denoting respect for elders in Indian culture.

Verma G was a third generation Indian Ayurvedic doctor who was initially taught by his grandfather, a very well-known Ayurvedic physician in Agra, India. Ayurveda, being one of the oldest medical systems in the world, was naturally passed down through generations. Verma G was always laughing or dancing, singing or chanting, and it seemed like no problem or discomfort was ever too complicated for him. There was always a simple solution for everything. He was so much fun to be around. He made the most delicious meals, and we used to make food and eat all together and dance on our summer holidays in Israel.

That summer, I had my first Ayurvedic consultation, and I will always remember that Verma G told me I was predominantly pitta dosha, which meant I had a lot of fire element in my body's constitution. He told me to take extra care in the summer season and to eat lots of cooling and refreshing foods, like watermelon and salads, and to drink a lot of water and fresh mint tea. He explained that it was very important that I eat on time (when I'm hungry), and that if I didn't, it could cause irritability and mood swings. With the help of my mum, we quickly adopted these suggestions, and before I knew it, I no longer got heat rashes, over-heated, or had irritable mood swings! From that moment onward, I was in awe of Ayurveda. How could it know me better than I knew myself?

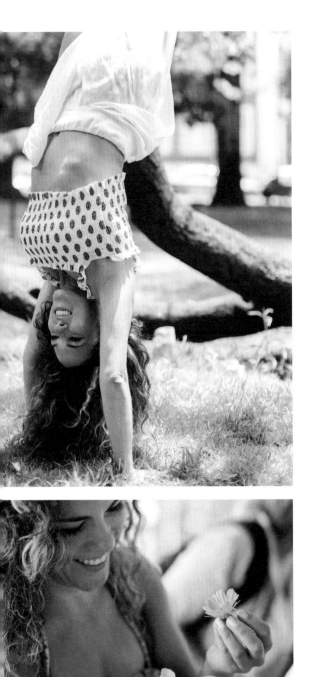

ANCIENT WISDOM + MODERN LIVING

Ayurvedic medicine quenched my thirst for understanding my body and gave me the tools to teach others how to understand theirs.

However, I was also eager to learn about the true effects of industrial modern food and chemicals on our body and planet. Ayurveda, being an ancient medicine and therefore created in a time when industrial food didn't exist, couldn't satisfy this hunger. So (after receiving my degree in Ayurveda) I moved to Florida and immersed myself in the world of modern science and nutrition at Hippocrates Health Institute, one of the leading institutes for reversing catastrophic disease. I wanted to learn the truth about food and vitality. In my gut I felt there was more truth to be discovered about the food industry, and I was ready to learn. I went on to research deeper into the relationship between food, health and vitality – and, above all, its relationship with our mood and thoughts.

BEFORE WE BEGIN

MY PHILOSOPHY

FOOD IS MEDICINE

"Let food be your medicine, and medicine be your food."

Hippocrates, the father of medicine

There's no doubt in my mind (and in Hippocrates' mind) that this is a fact. However, long-lasting health begins in the mind. Then everything else is effortless.

Somehow, losing the capacity to see details allowed me to see the bigger picture. Rather than focusing on what I couldn't see, I started to see life in a different light and from a different perspective, with form, colour and feeling. When we focus on the form, details are far less important. This is the foundation of my philosophy – because the way you think is important, before you fill in the content.

I couldn't let my eyesight limit me.

What limits us the most nowadays is our mind – the foundation that culminates in our actions and choices. By changing, unblocking, removing the limits from our minds, thoughts and imagination, we are giving ourselves a new chance of life. A new opportunity to live freely and unbound. A chance to build a life you love.

Health and wellness is not always about eating well and going to the gym. It's about your mindset and how you think. How we think influences every choice we make.

My approach to vitality is not a diet. It is a state of being, a mindset for a positive and sustainable way of life. I call it **MorLife Wellness.** It's for anyone interested in living out the best version of themselves, preventing disease, or building a life that they choose and really love living.

MorLife Wellness opens up a world of vitality. It's a practical, fun approach to healthy living for busy minds. This lifestyle opens up an undiscovered world of flavours, colours, new ingredients, perspectives and thought pathways that make life a whole lot more fun! There is nothing better than feeling truly amazing from the inside out!

This approach understands that the way you think influences how you eat and live. Our mindset is closely related to our daily choices; it's pretty impossible to try and change our habits without addressing our mindset. My philosophy starts in our head (mind) and then flows naturally into our body and life. We don't talk about good and bad foods, rather we dive into knowledge, facts and fun, trying to understand as we create new perspectives. **When you change your perspective, there's a sense of freedom, space and empowerment.** We create new pathways and new relationships to everything around us. It's rather magnificent! Sometimes a single conversation can refresh your perspective in brilliant ways. MorLife Wellness aims to inspire and create new perspectives that enhance your life without calorie counting, restrictions, or stress.

We will explore different levels of nourishment, some of which are not edible – one of my favourite principles that has changed my relationship with food forever.

A LIFESTYLE, NOT A RELIGION

Health, vitality, food choices, and lifestyle habits are not a religion. When it comes to our food and lifestyle, nothing can be set in stone. The way you choose to live your life can evolve and accompany your state of being at every moment. There is an increasing number of "diets" or ways to eat: vegan, vegetarian, keto, paleo, breatharian… It can feel like you have to make a choice and stick to it. You don't.

CREATING HABITS

Diets don't work. Research shows that we might be enthusiastic for the first week or two, but sooner or later, we all return to our old habits. People who go on a diet often regain more weight than they lost in the first place.

The first secret to succeed in creating new habits is overcoming the challenge in finding better alternatives to what we're used to. The second secret is to keep things simple and basic.

The best way to change a habit is to change your perspective, the foundation on which everything roots from. Change your perspective, change your life.

Everything new is strange at first, but we are creatures of habit. Once your mind becomes accustomed to the new habit it no longer finds it strange. We've created a new neural pathway.

Take sexy small steps – they often lead to the best outcomes. Where change comes gradually and naturally it is far more likely to become a habit, rather than trying to enforce too many changes over a short space of time. The smaller and easier the change, the more likely it is that it will stick. Changes don't have to be drastic or expensive, as this book will show you! **Sometimes the smallest step in the right direction ends up being the biggest step of your life.**

MY APPROACH, MY MANTRAS

Along my journey, I created three mantras that are embedded in MorLife Wellness and this book!

MANTRA #1
Life is a joy.

Life is a joy. Everything we do should be executed with a sense of joy. Anything that takes the joy from life should be paused, rethought, and done differently.

The joy of eating, thinking, dancing, sleeping and being are all part of MorLife Wellness, which gives us the strength to make the best of our journey. Even when things suck and challenges arise, joy makes the ride so much better!

MANTRA #2
Food must taste absolutely delicious and wonderful, no matter what.

As a nutrition specialist and health educator, I have never, nor will I ever, compromise flavour or the joy of eating for the idea of health. It doesn't make sense. In fact, the foundation of proper digestion in Ayurvedic medicine is based on pleasing the senses. Eating tasteless food just because it's "healthy" can result in indigestion and malabsorption.

MANTRA #3
It only works when you make it work for you.

Things need to be do-able, simple, easy and fun, so you're likely to repeat them day after day.

Whatever diet or lifestyle changes you want to make, if they don't fit into your current lifestyle then you're not likely to make those changes. I learned this first hand. I tried to begin regular yoga classes at

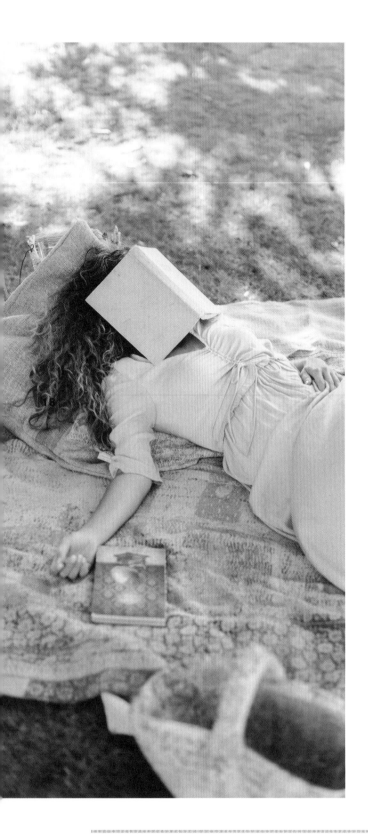

5.30pm every day, but I was never really ready to leave the office to get there on time. It was just too early and so I never made it. Instead of trying to change my whole life at once, I accepted that I like working around 5pm. So, I looked at what is realistic and realized that I need to find a yoga class that fits into my schedule – rather than trying to change my life or schedule to fit around yoga.

My mum was one of my first clients when I was still at university. What she does in one day we all do in a week. It was impossible to fit anything into her schedule. I had to create a healthy lifestyle that fitted into her over-booked schedule. This was a great challenge and an opportunity to practise and learn. It is evident that the only way someone can ever implement a better habit is if it can practically fit into their lifestyle. I learned quickly that the best approach was the one you're going to do. And the only way to make real changes is to start small and take it easy on yourself. In fact, the best outcomes are often full of slow, steady change and transformation.

WHY I DECIDED TO WRITE THIS BOOK

> "This may be the first generation in history to die before their parents."
>
> *Brian Clement, PhD, Hippocrates Health Institute*

I wrote this book because we have the right to the truth, nothing but the truth. But somehow we don't have access to it. We have become disconnected to the basics in life. If electricity stops tomorrow, we are all doomed. If I handed you a bag of seeds because that was all there was to survive, I think it's safe to say that we would all be screwed. Most of us don't know where our liver is, why our minds don't stop, or what it means when our stomach hurts. We have lost our innate capacity to care for ourselves. I've met so many people that want to feel better, but they don't know how. They're off spending tons of money trying to buy healthier products, but fooled by health marketing. I've seen too many people lose their life at too young an age to diseases that are curable and preventable. I've met so many children and young adults who have lost their quality of life to conditions that are reversible. This doesn't make sense. We don't need to constantly suffer unnecessarily. Too many of us have accepted physical and mental discomforts as common day-to-day conditions.

If so many diseases are preventable and even curable, why don't we know how to prevent them? **Why is knowledge used as power in our industry to keep people ignorant so that we simply can't do it better? Knowledge has taught me that we are the only people responsible for our health.** The medical model of our current society has become a business more than a service. Just like in any business the main goal is profit. There is no monetary gain in teaching you to prevent disease, if the main way the industry makes money is when people are sick.

My first client once I returned to Portugal after specializing at the Hippocrates Health Institute was a lovely man called Joao. To his surprise and my delight Joao reversed type 2 diabetes in three weeks! As much as I believed everything I was studying was possible and true, it became far more realistic when I started seeing my own clients manifesting miraculous change before my very eyes. There's nothing more rewarding than seeing your client return after only seven days of making small steps in their diet or lifestyle with less pain, less swelling and feeling more vibrant, confident and happy in their body and life. Clients kept coming, eager to learn a new paradigm on disease and discomfort.

One of my clients, Sandra, was suffering from rheumatoid arthritis. We began to treat her swelling and excruciating pain that came with it. Sandra came back ecstatic, as she could see her wrist bone after cutting the crap for just six days. Her systemic and joint pains had decreased drastically and she no longer suffered from an over bloated stomach. She continues to reap the benefits of living in harmony with her own body and nature.

MY MISSION

This book is one step towards my mission of creating a like-minded community of the coolest people ever – free from chronic disease and discomfort, confident, connected and at peace in their body; people that live in harmony with themselves and nature. Inspired by knowledge, empowered by courage, and fuelled by joy. A community that shines bright from the inside out with more life.

Only with knowledge and awareness can we make any real choices for ourselves, our families and our children.

I'm so excited to begin this journey with you. The chapters to come will take you on a journey towards vitality, joy and a lot of boogying, and feeling more alive! We address every aspect needed to fully develop the tools and resources you need to get connected and live better. From re-establishing communication with your body, understanding food on an essential level and how daily food choices also affect our planet's health, to exciting concepts that changed my life, understanding our mind, rocking ancient wisdom and the courage needed to shine bright and be yourself!

I'd love to connect and hear from you on this journey! Find me on danahmor.com – I can't wait!

HOW TO READ THIS BOOK

Each chapter could be a book in its own right, but I didn't want you walking around with 14 books! So I simplified and fine-tuned every chapter so that a complete life coaching kit could fit into a single book. A book that could accompany you on every step of your journey. Every chapter has a practical section. If you're in the mood to get down, jump to the practical section to get going, and read the whys later. Read it in whichever order you choose. Read the chapter that attracts you most, make it work for you (Mantra #3). You make the rules. You da boss!

Before we get started there's just one rule: **Do not stress-out, no matter how bad it seems.** There is always a fun, adventurous solution.

Stress is by far one of the most toxic chemicals on earth. So, put on some music, do a little dance, sing, laugh, but please don't stress. Be gentle with yourself. Aim for joy and **not perfection**. Perfection is a dangerous illusion – it doesn't exist and usually causes you to give up. See everything as an adventure and a process. We learn by listening to our body and accepting with trust that our body knows best, because it does. **Your willingness is your strongest asset. Never give up or lose your will to try again. Smile even if it sucks, light a candle, watch the sun set, and remember tomorrow is a new day! Enjoy and don't take me too seriously.**

With warm hugs and a big smile,

Danah ♡

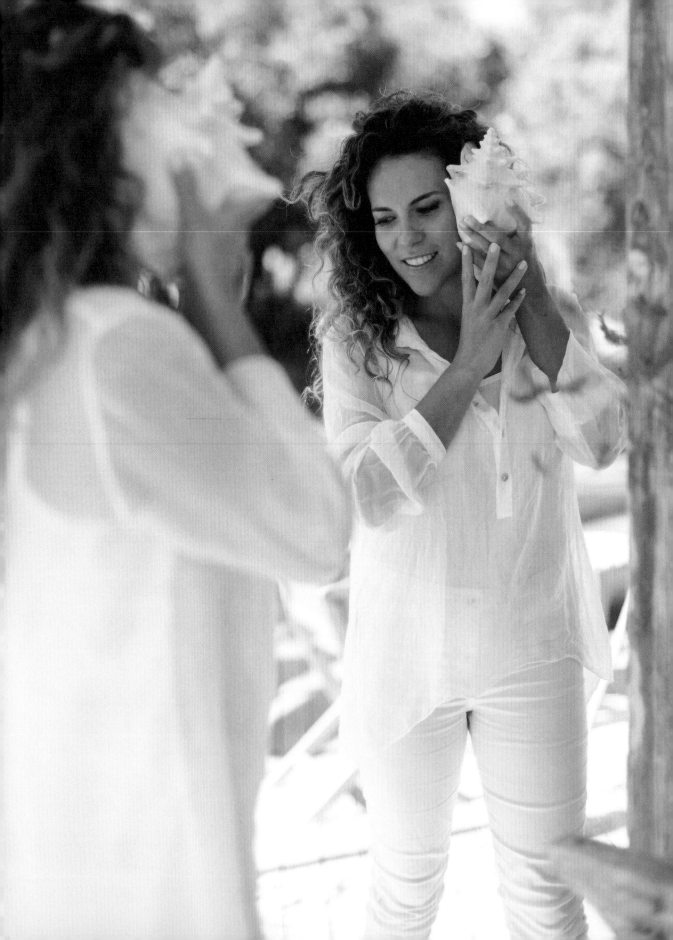

Listen to your body; it's trying to tell you something nobody else can.

Chapter 1

LISTEN TO YOUR BODY

QUESTION WHAT YOU ARE TOLD

NUTRITION IS ONE OF THE MOST CONFUSING TOPICS TODAY. THERE ARE STUDIES SHOWING THE OPPOSITE OF WHAT WE THOUGHT TO BE TRUE ABOUT FOOD. FOR EXAMPLE, WE'VE LONG THOUGHT THAT MILK IS ESSENTIAL FOR HEALTH. BUT THERE ARE NOW SEVERAL STUDIES THAT SUGGEST MILK CAN BE HARMFUL TO OUR VITALITY.

As research has developed, scientific papers have been published that suggest that milk isn't in fact essential to our diet. So how are we supposed to know what's the truth?

If we want the science behind something, we must look at the studies and understand who funded them. Real research is highly expensive so it's hard to fund research that is not linked to a consequent income through sales. Naturally, if there is research, someone paid for it. Unless it's funded by a neutral, unbiased party, it could be considered mis/disinformation. Most companies research something with the objective of making a profit.

Unfortunately, there is a lot of financial interest behind scientific studies, and the industry has pushed for studies to be published that show we need certain foods in our diet, even if it's not exactly true.

"It is simply no longer possible to believe much of the clinical research that is published."

Dr Marcia Angell, physician and longtime Editor-in-Chief of the New England Journal of Medicine

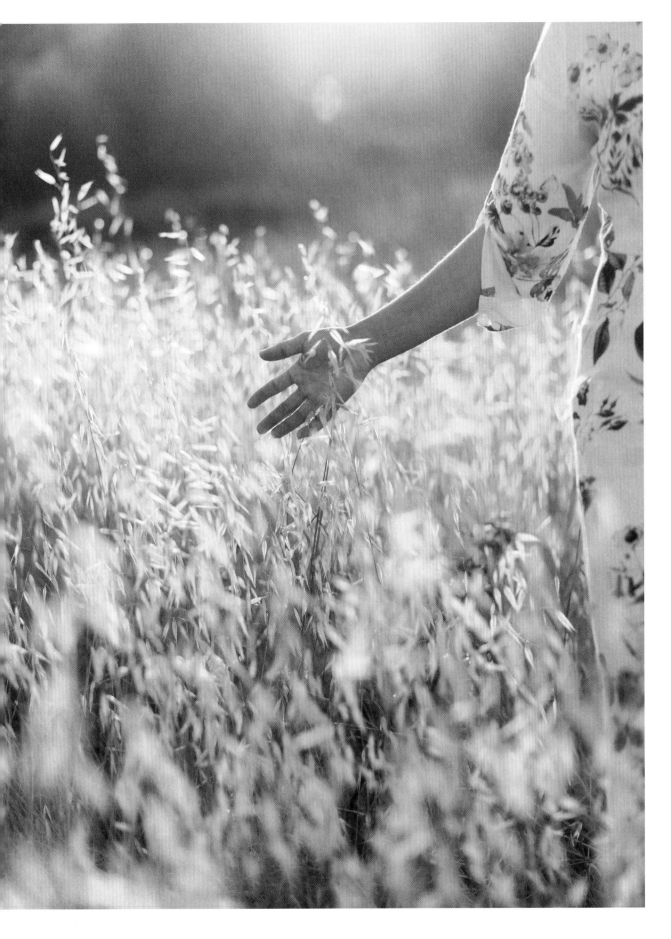

NO FOOD IS FORBIDDEN, UNLESS YOUR BODY SAYS SO

When it comes to nutrition and our health, I like to keep it as simple as possible, to understand the science and the facts, and then make my own conclusions by listening to my body when it reacts with foods or chemicals.

There is no forbidden food, unless your body says so. We can eat anything we want as long as our bodies agree. We just need to learn to understand how our bodies communicate. **The secret to vitality is not being obsessed with what you eat or how often you exercise. It's about getting in tune with yourself and your environment.** Most of us are so disconnected from ourselves and nature that we don't recognize a stomach ache as the body signaling a problem, we don't know what vegetables grow in which season, how milk or meat really gets into our supermarket, or where our liver is located.

We need to re-tune our mindset and understand that we are an expression from the inside out and not from the outside in. If our mindset is in tune with nature, we naturally make new choices without feeling restricted. Changing the way we think is the only way we can positively change our lives. When we change our perspective, we suddenly have new desires, different cravings; we no longer want the same things, and making positive choices becomes effortless. I've lived through this, and I can tell you how much better it is than forcing a new diet or lifestyle upon yourself. We might have to put in a bit of effort to achieve a new way of thinking, a new mindset, but then it becomes natural, even fun.

If your mindset is in harmony with your essence, you will make new choices naturally without having to sacrifice what you think you need. Instead, you choose what you want.

"When I changed my mindset from 'I can't eat that' to 'I don't want to eat that', I felt empowered and strong. I was no longer a victim to my thoughts."
Gal, 22, political sciences student, Paris

How do we know what we truly want? The connection between our body and our spirit is the foundation of life. Our mindset can allow or interfere with this connection. When our personality is in alignment with our spirit, that is authentic empowerment. The capacity to listen and foster the connection between these two is a secret for true inner joy and happiness.

WHEN DID WE STOP LISTENING?

I have always heard a clear voice in me that sounded humble, generous and real. Then all the other voices invaded my head – what my parents, teachers, sports coaches, and anyone that came into my life thought they should tell me about how to live or even how to listen to myself. Now it's hard to know which voice is really me. It may be the hardest thing to re-learn, because so much noise has invaded our bodies that it can be hard to know when it's really us speaking. But taking care of our body relies on our ability to listen to ourselves.

When I was studying Ayurvedic medicine at university in London, we were constantly reminded that our modern medical system separates the body from the mind (forget the spirit). In Ayurvedic medicine, the body, mind and spirit are inter-connected. How you think and express yourself is reflected in your physical body. How you eat and act is reflected in your spirit and mood. Ideally your spirit should shine and be expressed all through your body and into your choices and actions. In every consultation with a client, I often speak about food last because, first of all, food isn't everything.

Awareness and knowledge are the basis of conscious choice-making. Without awareness and the capacity to think, question, reflect, and make our choices, are we any more than puppets?

The decisions you make and actions you take are the means by which you evolve. Each moment, you choose the intentions that will shape your experiences and where you focus your attention.

ANCIENT WISDOM

I'm so excited to share a drop of the wisdom and knowledge of Ayurveda with you, one of the oldest medical systems that exists. Ayurveda, the science of life, introduced me to a world I didn't know existed; a world of peace and harmony for health and vitality. It is far more appealing to me than the Western medical and nutritional world that seems so obsessive.

Ayurveda gave me insight and knowledge that allowed me to see and understand life from a point of view that simplifies and answers so many questions. Considered the mother of medicine, Ayurveda is more than 10,000 years old. It's a holistic science that takes the whole person into consideration: body, mind and spirit. Every part of our body is connected. Our thoughts and emotions can affect our digestion, just as our physical sensations can affect our mind. If everything is interconnected, our bodies can constantly speak to us through physical signs. It was through the study of Ayurvedic medicine that I learned how important it is to listen to my body, especially when it comes to food,

digestion and lifestyle – and how I understood the connection between food and mood. Ayurveda celebrates our bio-individuality, that everybody is unique, so we have to learn what diet and lifestyle best fits us.

So, the real secret to vitality is understanding your body's language and improving your communication with it – on every level.

DECODING THE EATING MECHANISM

Signals of hunger and thirst are often mixed; we can feel hungry when in fact our body is trying to tell us that we need water. The differences between feelings of hunger and pure boredom are foggy. Not to mention, we neglect most serious signs of congestion or inflammation (especially in our gut and brain). Most of us have lost connection and communication with our body. Some of us use alcohol, coffee, painkillers or other substances like sugar to numb our body's signs and symptoms.

How many of us understand our own body's language? Do we eat to live, or because we're hungry, bored

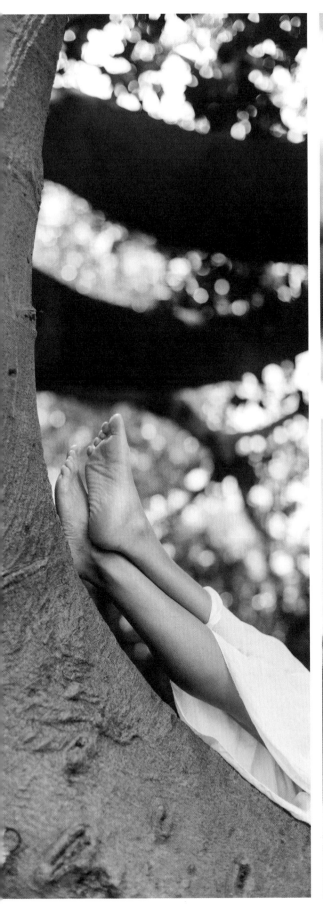
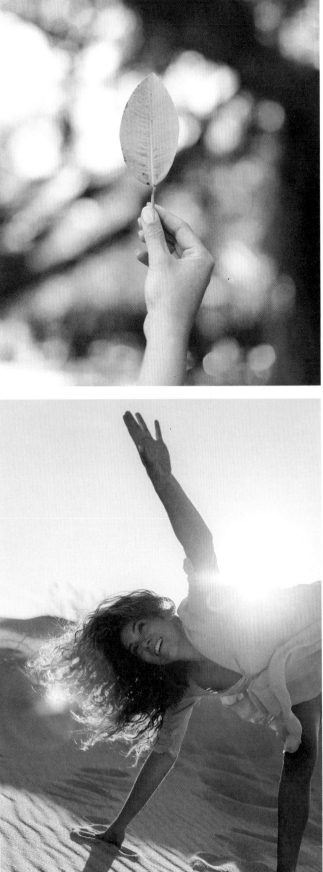

or lonely? Have you ever thought about why you are eating? When you eat, are you eating because you are hungry and want to nourish your mind and body? Are your eating habits no longer triggered by internal necessity, but rather by external factors?

Time: who decides when we are hungry?

How often do we eat because the time says so? It's dinner time, or snack time. Next time you eat, ask yourself beforehand, "Am I really hungry? Do I need to eat right now?"

Reason: hungry, thirsty, lonely, or bored?

How often do we look for food because we're bored or lonely? (I know I often found myself looking to munch on something when I was bored of studying.) Research suggests that 50 per cent of people open the fridge, look inside, and then close it when they arrive home. (Interesting. What are we looking for?)

What are you hungry for? Just because you feel like eating doesn't always mean you're actually hungry. I call this appetite. If you pay attention, these moments of "emptiness" can come from a lack of fulfillment in another area of your life that you're neglecting. (It's not all

about food). Next time you reach for food when you've already eaten and should feel satisfied, ask yourself, "What am I hungry for?" (Go for a walk, call a friend, or write a book!)

Are you thirsty? Hunger and thirst trigger the same hormonal mechanism. Next time you're hungry, drink water!

Quantity: who decides?

Who or what tells us to stop eating? Is it the size of our plate, our stomach–brain communication, the moment we finish tasting everything at the buffet, or the moment we are about to burst?

Satiety, the feeling of being full, takes 20 minutes to kick in. If you gobble down food too quickly, not only can you get indigestion but you'll probably eat too much food. Slow down when you eat. Put your fork and knife down between bites while you chew – this works really well! Chew your food so well that it's liquid when you swallow. Appreciate the food you're eating, where it came from, how it grew. Notice what you eat, and chill out when you eat so that you can hear your body telling you, "That's enough, thank you!" You may notice that you're full before you expect. Ideally we should stop eating just before we're full for the best digestion (This is also a winner for weight management!).

Creating a ritual around our meals and snacks also helps our mind focus on what we are doing – in this case, eating. For example, if we are trying to eat while having an overly animated conversation, this could keep us from staying connected to the body. Watching TV, reading a book or any other activity are all distractions. Next time you eat, simply focus on the smell, the taste and the texture of the food you eat. Notice what textures and flavours you enjoy. Is the food the right temperature? Put down your fork between bites, and focus on chewing. And don't forget to breathe. Breathing while you eat (through your nose, of course!) is another great way to slow yourself down at meal times and re-connect to your body. Even taking a few breaths before you start eating can help prepare your body for digestion, putting you in "rest and digest" mode.

BODY LANGUAGE AND SIGNALS

How often do we read our body's signals without the mind interfering, ignoring or distorting?

If your car is giving a red alert signal, but you don't stop to work out what the alert is for, what happens? It's likely your car doesn't last long.

Smoke signals from our bodies mean, "Please do something different because something is wrong!" If you ignore those mild smoke signals, a fire could be just up ahead.

Check out the guidelines in the table on the following page. You can create some for yourself too!

|31|

HOW SERIOUS ARE YOUR SIGNALS

YELLOW ALERT	ORANGE ALERT	RED ALERT
An occasional mild pain/ discomfort, indigestion, or headache.	Medium pain, heartburn, indigestion, bloating and rashes. All mild, acute discomforts or yellow alerts that repeat themselves frequently including general discomfort/ pain, headaches, bloating, acid reflux and constipation are orange alerts.	Continuous repeated and regular orange alerts. When orange alerts become regular or chronic, they are red alerts, and if ignored or symptomatically treated, these mild symptoms can lead to serious long-term complications or disease. For example, chronic constipation can lead to intestinal cancer and other intestinal complications. Uncontrolled heartburn can lead to throat, voice and dental problems, as well as asthma and other respiratory complications, if not worse conditions.

YELLOW ALERTS:
This discomfort is occasional, which means it happens a few times a year – not more. If you think, you can probably connect it to some sort of event like eating bad food which causes a stomach ache, a sleepless night leading to a headache or eating something that caused heartburn.

ORANGE-TO-RED ALERTS:
The difference between a yellow and orange alert is the level of pain and/ or the fact that it is repetitive.

The reoccurring discomfort is indicating something continues to be wrong and needs attention, not symptomatic relief. When yellow signals occur every month, and even more than once a month they become orange and could even become red alerts if they are not tended to. At this point we need to stop, look and listen to what we have done differently. Looking at internal and external factors will help us scan different areas of our lives.

RESPONDING TO THE NEED

Responding to these symptoms does not mean numbing them with symptomatic relief, like a painkiller. Your body is telling you something is wrong, so please try something different. For example, if your stomach hurts after eating something, try eating differently or different foods. If you have headaches, drink more water, or is there something in particular that is causing you stress? Try to relax more, exercise and spend more time in nature... it's simple; just try anything different in a better direction.

Next time you feel discomfort, ask yourself if there have been any changes in your diet, activities, emotions and sleep. For example:

* *What did I do differently today, yesterday, this week?*
* *Have I had enough water?*
* *Did I get upset or angry?*
* *When did this discomfort begin? What has happened since then?*
* *What have I eaten in the last few days? Anything different?*
* *Is this reoccurring? If so, try to notice what happened around these discomforts*
* *Does it happen after a particular meal? Does it happen after an argument with your spouse? Does it happen when you stress at work, with the kids? Does it happen in the evening or morning? What happens around that time?*
* *How did I feel? What were my thoughts about?*
* *What did I eat? What did I drink?*

Most discomforts are triggered by emotional or/and physical events. By understanding the trigger, we can prevent the discomfort. For example, I have always loved homemade desserts, but I've linked them to my allergies. So I started experimenting and found that if I eat ice cream before 6pm I have no allergenic response. This could be related to the fact that my body has time to process the sugar before I sleep and therefore it doesn't affect my system the following day.

If you are eating something that is irritating your system and causing you discomfort as a result, this can be solved simply. Becoming more aware of how you feel after your meals, interactions etc., and figuring out if you feel better when you don't eat a certain food, is how you begin a conversation with your body. Becoming aware of our signals, responding and experimenting is crucial to reconnect and communicate with ourselves.

I sometimes get headaches. At first I asked myself if I'd had enough water that day, and I made an effort to drink more. I noticed that drinking water often helped the headache go away. But I started to get a stronger type of headache. By questioning what happens around these headaches that may be causing the discomfort, I realized they always occurred before or on a very stressful day or event. I realized that my headaches were related to my anticipation of stress. I was stressing about what was to come, that hadn't even happened yet. I was thinking too much, and all my energy was getting stuck in my head. Now that I know that too much thinking/stressing causes my headaches, when I start to feel a headache coming on, I can prevent it by trying to calm my mind down and stop any recurrent thoughts.

My client Michael came to see me when he had already made a connection with his symptoms. His mouth was filled with sores for years and he was overweight and always bloated. He heard about gluten and dairy sensitivities and experimented one day. He stopped consuming dairy at first. He noticed after two days that the sores in his mouth had disappeared. This is a great example of body connection – because he felt discomfort and acted upon it. He tried something different. By trying something different he discovered his body didn't agree with dairy. He stopped consuming it and his discomfort vanished. After a few weeks his belt size reduced by six holes! He was shocked. Michael never thought that one type of food – and something he had been brought up to believe was healthy – could cause so much discomfort.

Maria decided to stop eating bread to lose weight. However, when she was on holiday she didn't mind and enjoyed bread as much as she wanted. She started to notice that on holiday she no longer had bowel movements, so she started to ask herself what she was doing differently. Firstly, she was on holiday, and she was more relaxed and less stressed, so emotionally it was positive. So she thought about food – how was her eating different? The only thing that was different was her bread consumption. She responded to the trigger and her constipation vanished. Now she enjoys her holidays much more without bread and no bloated abdomen!

Often the idea of having to give up certain foods is outweighed by the comfort we feel once we free our bodies from the discomfort.

As I have said before, there's nothing more addictive than feeling amazing! Asking ourselves the right questions will lead us to an answer, a choice and an action.

IS TRUST THE BRIDGE BETWEEN LISTENING AND ACTING?

When we feel or hear something inside, many of us don't trust enough to truly listen and follow through with action. As if there's a resistance, a doubt. Our body is communicating and if we don't listen with trust, we may fail to respond to the necessity of what is needed at that moment. Rather, we ignore it and move on, as most of us do.

This happens in our relationships with food, with people and with ourselves as we focus on our external life and society's expectations.

Our body always gives us feedback, and this goes for everything: eating a certain food; hanging out with a certain person; working a certain job; and so on. If we don't listen with trust, we ignore our body's wisdom and continue to engage in harmful relationships. **Trust is essential when we listen to our body – without it, we have no consequent action.**

The interest and willingness to want to understand the body better is a trigger to becoming more aware. When you want to become more aware, you start to notice things you never noticed. When we begin to listen more carefully to our body, our body starts to speak more clearly. It's a channel of communication that has to be rekindled and empowered.

When I first started losing my eye sight, it was harder because I didn't trust. As I learned to listen to myself, and trust more, I found that this inner communication became stronger. The more I listened, the more my body spoke.

There are many things we may want to adapt and change on our path, and this mustn't be frightening but, rather, exciting because only with groovy changes and decisions can we create a life we choose and love.

Listening is a journey that can only help you evolve and foster a magnificent life. It all starts by listening to your body.

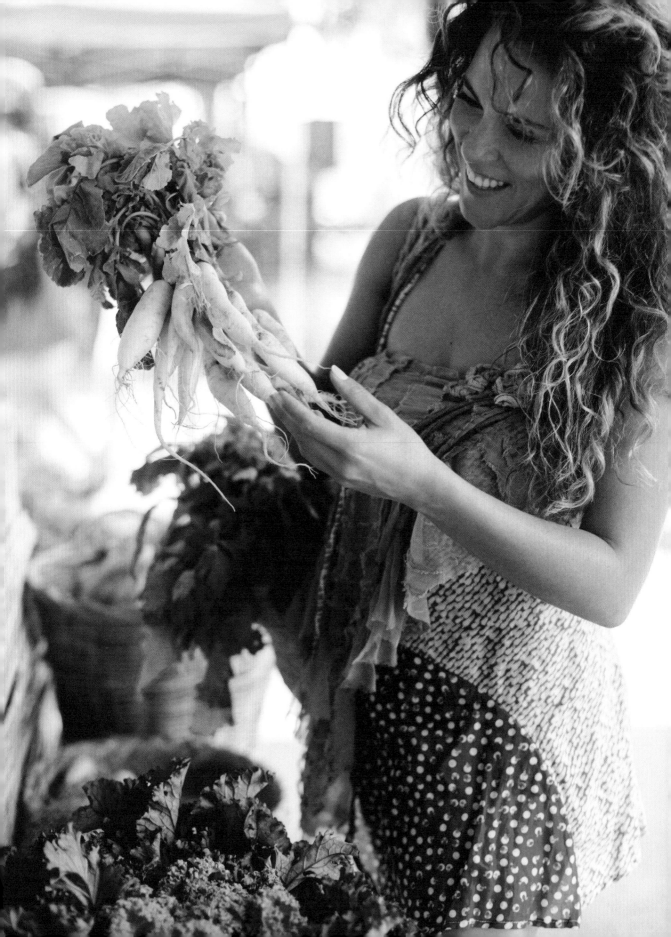

Many of us spend more time shopping for shoes and cars than we do for our own health. When it comes to food be as picky as you are with buying a car or shopping for shoes!

Chapter 2

LOVE REAL FOOD – A FOOD REALITY CHECK

WHAT'S ALL THE FUSS ABOUT?

"MY GRANDPARENTS ATE IT AND THEY WERE FINE, SO WHY CAN'T WE JUST EAT AS THEY DID? WHAT'S THE PROBLEM?"

I GET ASKED THIS QUESTION A LOT. THE FOOD INDUSTRY HAS CHANGED SINCE OUR GRANDPARENTS' TIME AND MUCH OF OUR FOOD NOW IS MASS PRODUCED (IN ENORMOUS FACTORIES), PROCESSED OR ALTERED IN SOME WAY FROM ITS NATURAL STATE.

In our modern industrial era of mass agriculture, factory farming and processed food, modern technologies and processes control our food system and interfere with its nutritional value.

Whether we eat it or not, we can all recognize junk food when we see it. We all know that junk food is unhealthy and highly processed. The trouble is that nowadays even food that we consider "real" food, such as milk, bread and meat, has been altered and denatured. It's shocking and hard to accept, but supermarkets sell products that look, taste and smell like food, but, in fact, should not be considered real food.

The challenge today is that most of us don't know how to tell the difference between a real natural food and an industrial artificial food.

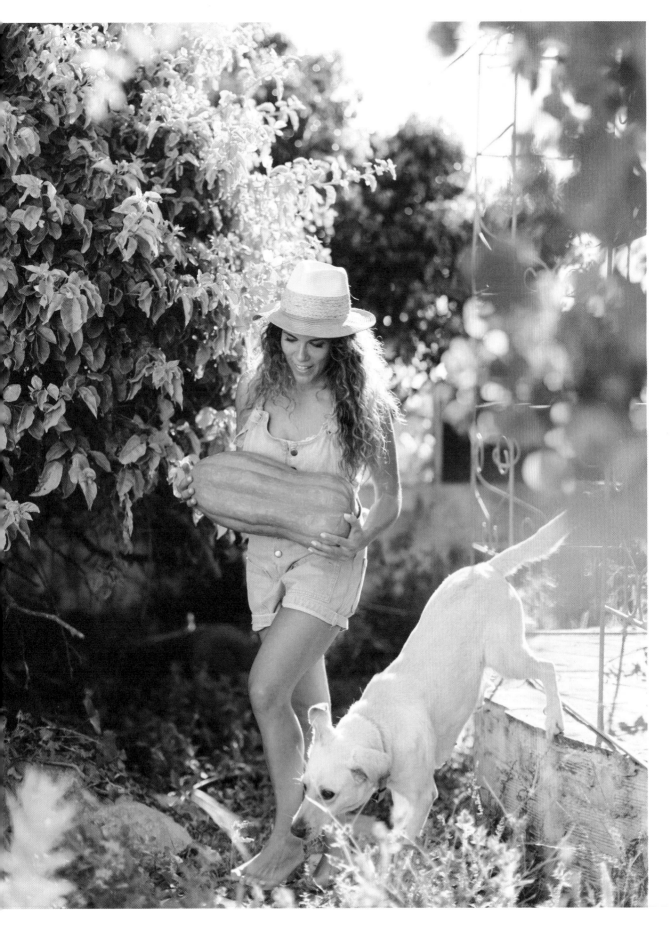

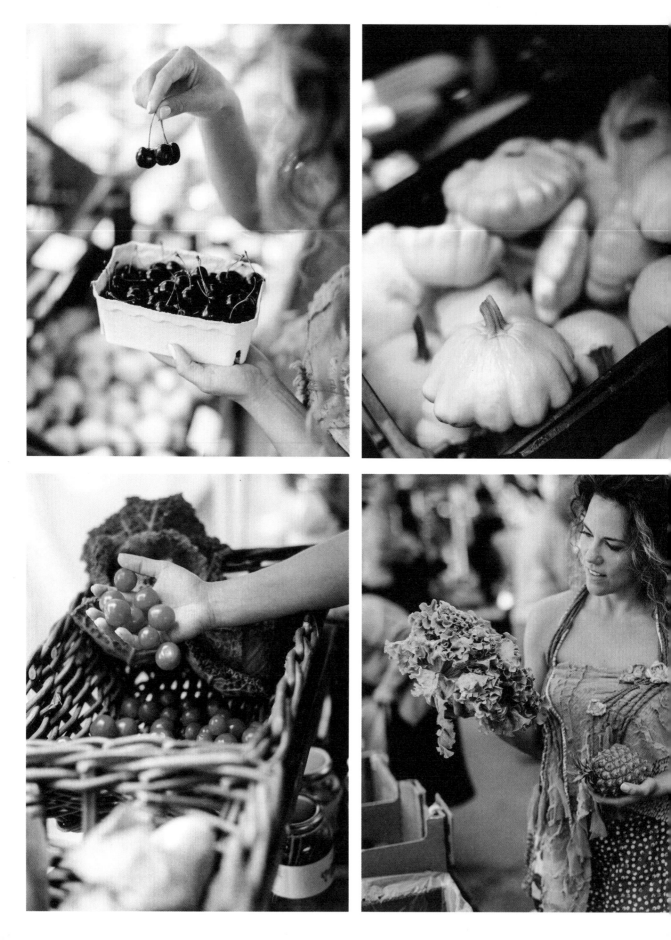

WHAT ACTUALLY IS REAL FOOD?

Real food is whole food, unprocessed, unrefined, not packaged or changed in any way from its natural state. Whole foods have no added ingredients like sugar, salt, vitamins, or any other artificial substances and additives. They are foods we can recognize straight from nature, like avocado, wholegrain rice, quinoa, pumpkin, beans and almonds.

No food is necessarily bad; it's what we have done to it that changes its nature and its effect on our bodies.

Love and eat real food as opposed to fake food. Today, we don't know what life was like before packaged food existed on the supermarket shelf. Loving real food is about learning to recognize real, natural, non-processed food from the stuff we are told is food.

WHAT ARE ARTIFICIAL PROCESSED FOODS?

Any food that has undergone a treatment or processing, even if it's just removing the shell from a grain, like white rice or white flour, makes it a refined, non-whole food. Every year, **70,000** new products are engineered and sold in the supermarkets. Most of these foods don't deserve to be called food. They're packaged and marketed with fancy colours so that they trigger our brain receptors for impulsive consumption. Not only are many of these foods products of a laboratory, they are highly addictive and packed with chemicals that damage our body so much that often toxins can't get out.

Food manufacturers use scientific research on how the brain reacts and responds to texture and taste, and how colours influence human emotion and behaviour, to stimulate our impulse to buy certain foods. This way they can guarantee that we will buy their products.

It has been proven that colour influences consumers not only on the conscious level but even on the subconscious level. Just to get an idea, research has shown that red is a powerful colour known to stimulate and excite, heighten nerve impulses and increase the heart rate. Red enhances the appetite and stimulates a physical response – impulse buying, for example.

Yellow is also an appetite stimulant. It makes people feel cheerful and optimistic. In fact, studies show that when we look at the colour yellow, our brain releases serotonin (the "feel good" chemical), which can make us feel good about what we are buying – even if it is junk.

Together, red and yellow evoke the taste buds and stimulate appetite. Now it's clear why this is a common choice in the fast food industry!

Industrialized fake foods can act like drugs in the body by causing the release of dopamine in our brain. They are addictive like drugs and are purposefully designed this way by food engineers so that we just keep eating more and more of these perfectly created money-making food-like substances.

Neuroscientist Dr Amy Reichelt explains that junk foods are refined in order to target our brain so that we lose control. This ensures that we will be coming back for more and more, which guarantees business and profits.

Industrialized artificial and fake foods are chemically engineered mixtures designed to play our brains so that we actually think we're eating highly nutritious food. Back in the day when we were hunter gatherers, food was scarce and our brains were designed to seek out high-calorie, salty, sweet or fatty foods as a survival mechanism. Nowadays, this no longer serves us, but our brains still work the same way.

Food companies therefore have highly skilled food engineers and neuroscientists working with them to design fake foods with exactly the right combination of sugar, salt and fat that stimulates our brain into producing pleasure chemicals like dopamine that quickly get us addicted and craving even more each time – just like a drug.

Fake foods attack our brain and nerve cells. Their consumption has been linked to depression, dementia, loss of memory, the incapacity to create new memories and several other mental disorders new to our generation.

Perhaps it all went wrong when the food sector – that should serve a nation – became an industry where profits and monetary goals have replaced service and quality.

FOOD INDUSTRY- DESIGNED FOR BUSINESS, NOT HEALTH

"Western diets now typically contain a toxic brew of synthetic chemicals that create hormonal imbalances, which result in food addictions and chronic illness."
Robert Lustig, Pediatric Endocrinologist

There are products on the shelf in our supermarkets that are seriously harmful. **Just like eating paint, it won't kill you if you do it once, but keep doing it and it will cause serious complications.** The food industry makes choices that harm our health and reduce the nutrient levels of food for profit and convenience.

The food industry is not always about feeding us or trying to keep people healthy. Mass production is a business and a very, very profitable one. The food industry makes choices with profits and convenience in mind, not the quality of food or our health, unfortunately. The processes that increase the shelf life of food, for example, strip it of nutrients, essential vitamins, minerals, fibre and everything good. We're basically eating calories with no nutrients.

When I started studying health and nutrition, I was shocked to discover that even foods I considered to be healthy were perfect examples of refined, un-whole, manipulated or contaminated food: yoghurt, muesli, oat bars, fish, healthy ready meals. Even supplements! Vitamin C (ascorbic acid) for example is synthetically and chemically created in a lab to mimic natural vitamin C. Most foods with health claims such as "fortified" or "diet" – even "natural" – written on them are usually packed with additives, chemicals or lab-produced vitamins. These pretend foods are far from anything we can consider natural or whole. **In fact, for a product to claim it is "natural", it only needs 10 per cent of its ingredients to be natural; it can be 90 per cent artificial and still claim to be natural!**

Commercial blueberries in muffins are made of petroleum; they are artificially coloured and flavoured to look and taste exactly like a blueberry, with a lengthy expiration date of four years. This is an example of the reality of common foods we eat every day scientifically engineered to look, taste, smell and feel like something they are far from being.

NOT-SO-REAL FOOD: ONCE NATURAL, NOW HIGHLY PROCESSED

Modern food is not created for human consumption. It's created for shelf life.

Chemically infused foods are engineered to create a similar effect to that of an orgasm in our brains, making them addictive no matter how bad they make you feel. Scientists have created toxic substances that are disguised as food, which when consumed are like a drug, causing a release of dopamine – which as we've seen will ensure you buy the product again and again. **Has the industry found a legal form of drug dealing where most of us are addicted drug users unknowingly?**

Industrial agriculture, factory farming, advanced food engineering, processing, and the increased usage of chemicals have disconnected us from our food and from nature. Most people today have little understanding of the concept of seasonal foods, how food grows or gets to their plates. We have everything in the supermarket all year round. It's a false concept of nature.

The industrialization and modernization of the food industry makes food more convenient. This convenience has increased quantity of production and reduced the quality and nutrient levels of food. These new foods, in colourful packaging, are easier to recognize as artificial or non-whole foods.

However, the real difficulty and saddest reality I've had to face so far has been learning how the foods our grandparents ate, which were once natural and whole, are now so highly processed they are better avoided altogether; they are some of the most allergenic and harmful foods today.

> "The food scientist's chemistry is designed to extend shelf life, make old food look fresher and more appetizing than it really is, and create an addictive relationship."
>
> *Alejandro Junger, author of* Clean

PROCESSING FOOD REDUCES NUTRIENT VALUE

From synthetic chemicals, processing, freezing, canning and refining, the food industry creates a degeneration in nutritional value of our food supply. The list below gives an idea of what nutrients are lost when we process foods, and why it's so much better to choose fresh options. Of course, if canned chickpeas are what makes it possible to make a quick hummus, rather than grabbing a burger, then canned chickpeas it is! But it's still important we're aware of what happens to our food when it's processed, pre-peeled, canned, frozen and pre-cooked.

Percentage of nutrients lost in processing methods:

Over-processing: 100%
Refining: 100%
Canning: 83%
Freezing: 50–80%
Drying: 30–80%
Cooking: 40–70%
Pasteurization: 50%
Early harvesting: 25%
Transporting: 25%
Storage: 25%

COOKING PRACTICES

When you are cooking veggies, try to lightly steam or steam fry them so they still retain some bite. This way they retain most of their nutrients. When we boil vegetables, many of the nutrients leach out into the water. If you drink the water or you're making a soup, that's great, but try not to throw out boiled vegetable water – it's full of nutrients! Food can lose up to 75 per cent of its nutrients to the water it's boiled in. Avoid microwaves because they reduce the nutrient content of your food.

MILK AND DAIRY - ONCE PURE, NOW INFLAMMATORY

We think of milk as a natural food from a cow, and yes, it used to be. However, when it became mass-produced, it became an industrialized food that no longer has the same nourishing qualities as it does in nature. When happy cows enjoy their life in a green field and provide milk to nourish their offspring, their milk is rich in nutrients, enzymes and probiotics. This natural milk from a happy grass-fed cow continues to be a whole food.

Nowadays, modern milk undergoes pasteurization and homogenization, which strip milk of its nutrients and nourishing enzymes. The process of removing fat or adding vitamins, minerals (fortified with synthetic calcium), sugar and even artificial flavours makes commercial milk a processed industrialized food. Milk is taken from cows that are impregnated solely for milk and veal production. At birth, the mother and baby are separated, and the calf has no right to its mother's milk, because this is now a business. In dairy factory farming, cows are artificially impregnated immediately after giving birth (with no break) and milked while pregnant. This means that our milk contains the hormones of a pregnant cow as well as all the chemicals injected into the mother cow.

Why do we drink milk? Is it because "it's full of calcium and therefore good for our bones"?

THE CALCIUM CONTROVERSY

Cows no longer feed in the sun on calcium-rich greens. This explains why their milk is no longer rich in calcium, and thus fortified with synthetic calcium. It is clear that the milk available in a supermarket is no longer a nourishing whole food. The consumption of commercial milk has been linked to acne, indigestion and many more discomforts. In fact, my first client solved his acne issues by ditching dairy altogether. He couldn't believe it.

WHEAT, BREAD AND ALL WHITE FLUFFY THINGS

"Wheat, or what we are being sold that is called 'wheat', is not really wheat at all but the transformed product of decades of genetic research aimed at increasing yield-per-acre."

William Davis, author of Wheat Belly

Modern wheat is quite different from what it used to be. The industrialization, mass production, cross-breeding, and advanced engineering over decades has transformed and altered the composition of modern wheat as well as the structure of gluten. The result is a genetically unique plant considerably shorter than real wheat with bigger seeds and higher yields.

The genetic difference between ancient wheat and modern wheat is more than the genetic difference between chimpanzees and humans, which is only one per cent! If we wouldn't mingle with a chimpanzee even if its genetic make-up is only one per cent different from ours, why are we fraternizing with genetically engineered wheat!

BREAD: A STAPLE FOOD TRANSFORMED INTO A NUTRITIONAL CATASTROPHE

Flour, yeast, water and salt are the traditional four ingredients of bread. Why then is our ordinary bread being infused with a long list of chemicals and additives? The industry is always pushing to make bread bigger, softer, cheaper, longer-lasting and seemingly healthier. What does this mean for us and our health?

Why mass production messed up bread for me

I love bread – the smell, the texture, the taste! But I cut it out of my diet ten years ago. After studying the details of mass baking, it made more sense to look for real-food options instead of what was being sold as healthy fresh bread.

INDUSTRIAL BREAD IS A MIXTURE OF:

1. Refined, nutrition-less, genetically engineered modern wheat flour.

2. Bleached flour that makes the bread whiter (purer-looking) and is devoid of natural nutrients that interfere with convenient mass baking.

3. Chemically created yeast that further irritates our intestines.

4. Hydrogenated fats (associated with heart disease) that improve bread volume, crumb softness and shelf life.

5. L-ascorbic acid (E300), a chemical which helps dough retain gas, making bread rise more, giving a false notion of value. This is also used in wholemeal bread!

6. L-cysteine hydrochloride (E920), soy flour, chemical emulsifiers and preservatives like calcium propionate.

Several agents, enzymes, additives and preservatives – in other words, harmful chemicals – are added to speed up dough rising times, increase volume, prolong shelf life, and make bread stay fluffy, soft and stretchy for longer and longer.

These additives improve the machinability of dough; they improve industrial procedures and mass factory baking so that **profits increase while our health declines.**

Even local bakers often use these additives and enzymes, unconsciously thinking they are improving their bread quality.

Try making your own bread. This way you'll know exactly what's in it. Simply slice it and freeze it so you always have healthy bread to hand.

HOLY BREAD TO CASH COW

Bread has been depicted by many religions as a holy symbol. In each part of the world, there is a traditional bread: mafra in Portugal, pita in the Middle East, chapati in India, to name a few. But because of its low ingredient costs, wheat has become a financial cash cow. With the low raw material cost, companies still receive endorsements to produce wheat. **Maybe this government money could go toward the growing of vegetables so they can be cheaper for the people!**

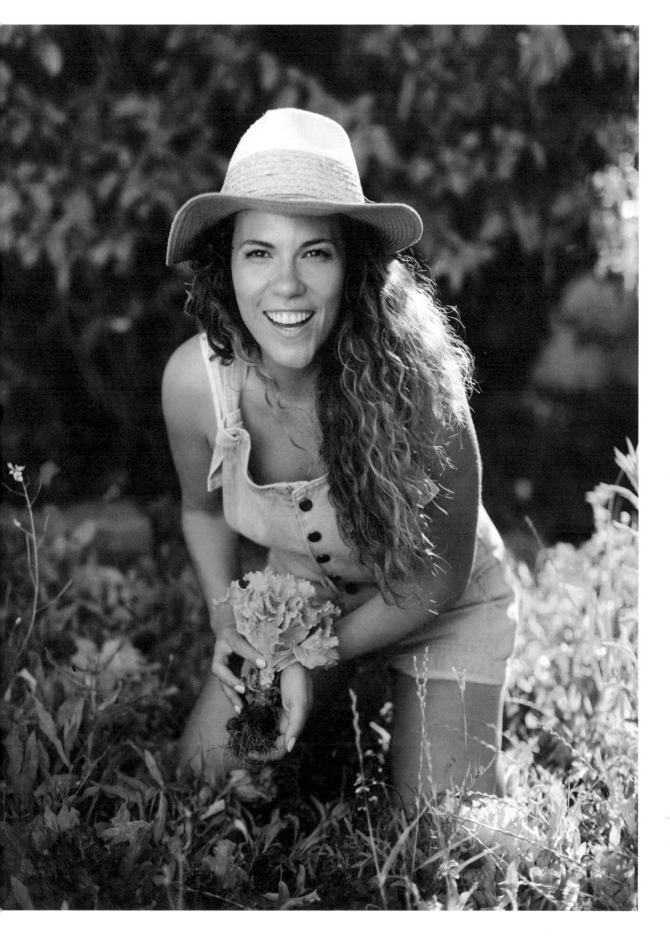

GMO: A BAD IDEA THAT'S GETTING WORSE

GMOs (genetically modified organisms) are plants or animals that have had their DNA modified.

WHY GENETIC ENGINEERING?

Plants are genetically modified to increase their production capacity for less money. Other reasons include becoming more resistant to environmental conditions like drought or pathogens, pesticides and insecticides. However, these GMOs may build up a resistance and then require even larger amounts of chemicals than before, which may be more harmful than helpful for our planet and bodies. This means that, eventually, we will be seeing more chemicals on our GMO crops, making them more toxic.

Genetic engineering began with the motivation to fight world hunger by increasing crop yields. So, if genetically engineered crops are cheaper to grow, have higher yields, and extend the time food remains edible, surely they mean more food for those who need it? The catch is that starvation and malnutrition is not about a lack of food in the world, but rather a problem of accessibility and distribution. **The paradox is that, currently, there are more obese people suffering from malnutrition than there are starving people in the world.** So, is the problem perhaps distribution and overfeeding rather than underfeeding?

CAN EATING GMO OR GE FOODS BE HARMFUL?

Genetic engineering began a long time ago. But it wasn't until recently that we started playing with the DNA of staple foods that have sustained generations, like grains. **Scientists now realize how much they don't know and that we, as a species, have entered one of the biggest scientific experiments** humanity has ever embarked upon. **Genetic modification and the effect of eating these foods has never been tested on a generation of humans and, therefore, cannot be considered safe, nor can its effects be known to us.** In short, we are the experimental guinea pigs of billion-dollar companies looking to make more billions by creating more food for less – and for most of us, it's costing us our vitality.

The changes and adulterations to our food and the pesticides sprayed onto our veggies have been linked to the rise of childhood diseases usually only found in adulthood, not to mention the increase in all forms of cancers.

The processes involved in genetically modifying the DNA of a unique species is very complicated because nature strives to protect the DNA of every species. Science currently uses a cell invasion technique with bacteria and viruses to get the genetic modification into the cell. **They create a parasitic event that breaks into the cell's DNA to change its natural coding so that it benefits the company's goals** – forget nature. Eeek!

GMOS AND HEALTH

Now that we can better see that our food supply is created with business in mind rather than health, this is the right moment to say that GMOs have not been proven safe, that testing has not been conducted for health purposes. With little to no regulating body in place, the GE companies conduct their own testing and report their own results to the government. But independent studies continue to show that GMO consumption can cause kidney, liver and reproductive problems and decrease immunity, among other issues.

GMO LABELLING: WHAT ARE WE EATING?

If someone is changing the nature of our food, **we have the right to know what we are eating**. Most of the GE firms are desperately trying to ban the need to label food that is genetically modified. Why? It's suspicious. GMO labelling is a big topic at the moment. Several countries around the world have compulsory GMO labelling, which has motivated companies to eliminate the use of GMO ingredients. Find out how you can help demand GMO labelling and make this obligatory worldwide!

The Environmental Working Group is an organization dedicated to protecting human health and the environment. Their team of scientists and experts make a huge effort to ensure someone is standing up for public health when government and industry won't. They educate and empower consumers to make safer and more informed decisions about the products they buy and the companies they support. In response to consumer pressure, companies are giving up potentially dangerous chemical ingredients in their products and improving their practices.

Join EWG's community and demand GMO labelling!

AVOID GE FOODS

Most corn, soybean, cotton, canola crops and sugar beans are now genetically modified. Unfortunately, with the lack of regulation around GMO labelling, it's hard to keep track. One or more of these GE foods can be found in almost every processed food. Keep up to date as new forms of GE foods are being launched into the market. Science is working on genetically modifying land animals and fish. GMO salmon is on the verge of being launched into the sea which could wipe out our natural wild species.

Four Simple Tips to Avoid GMOs:

1. Buy certified organic products because they cannot knowingly contain GMO ingredients.

2. Look for NON-GMO Project verified logos.

3. Avoid ingredients at risk of GMO like soy-bean products, corn, papaya, canola, cottonseed, and sugar from sugar beans – if it is not pure cane sugar then it probably has GMO ingredients.

4. Join a community that raises awareness about GMO foods to stay informed and up to date.

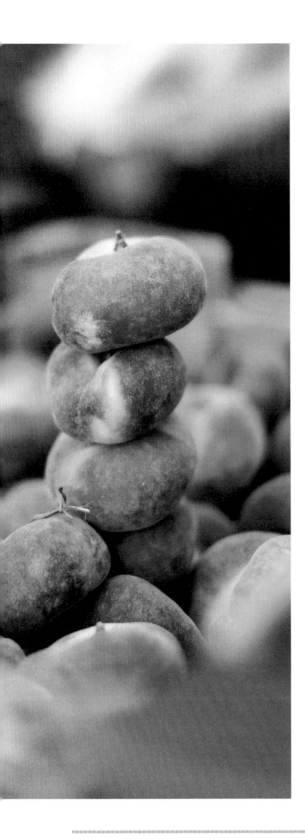

SOY

The story of soy is similar to that of margarine – it's heavily marketed as a health food while perhaps causing more harm than good. I meet so many people that strive to be healthy, buying soy products at higher prices when it could be harming their bodies.

Soy is a controversial topic with studies showing health benefits for and against it. In the case of soy, the problem isn't only the bean, it's what we do to the bean. Soy is so highly processed and genetically engineered that I prefer to avoid it all together.

|53|

Soy facts

Soy is the hardest to digest of all the beans. The health claims made about soy are based on Eastern cultures that eat only fermented soy like miso, tempeh, tamari and some tofu. Fermentation neutralizes the toxins in soybeans, cultures healthy probiotics, and can be beneficial to health when properly made. Asians consume soy foods in small amounts as a condiment, not as a replacement for animal foods. The colourful packaging of modern soy foods like yogurt, ice cream, snacks, and pretend meat and cheese, are not healthy nor real forms of food. In fact, they are highly processed fake foods, rich in toxins, fake flavours, additives and harmful chemicals.

Many of us eat soy every day, and we don't even know it.

Soy is one of the cheapest crops on the planet, so the industry has found ways to use every part of the bean for profit. Soy is often marketed on our cereal boxes as the star health-promoting ingredient and is hidden in more than 60 per cent of processed packaged foods.

Soy oil is the base for most vegetable oils. Soy lecithin, the waste product left over after the soybean is processed, is used as an emulsifier. Since it's cheaper than any other crop, soy flour appears in baked and packaged foods because it secretly reduces costs. Soy is even added to hamburgers and injected under poultry skin to increase bulk and reduce costs.

Soy can be found in:

noodles
cookies
wholegrain crackers
burgers
gummy bears
sauces
fast food
canned tuna
soups
breads
meat
chocolate

Ground beef for school children can contain up to 30 per cent soy. Food served to prisoners can contain up to 70 per cent soy. Eek!
Soy protein is isolated and added into any processed food to claim it is "high in protein".

This is not real food.

"Soy protein isolate was invented for use in cardboard. It hasn't actually been approved as a food ingredient."

Kaayla Daniel, The Dark Side of Soy

Just so we get the idea, soy is so cheap that it's even being used in non-food products like home and car foam insulation, cardboard adhesive, crayons, bio diesel, wax, fertilizer, fungicide, candles, plastic cloth fibres and insecticides.

It's even hidden in pet food and body-care products.

Soy has natural toxins

Soybeans naturally contain toxic substances and antinutrients. When we eat soy products we consume its toxins as well. Toxins and antinutrients include oxalic acid and phytates, potent enzyme inhibitors, and thyroid-suppressing compounds. Although these sound intergalactic, they are ingredients to avoid. These substances are harmful and interfere with the body's ability to properly function.

Soy is in fact listed on the poisonous plant database. Four countries warn parents not to feed soy to their babies: Germany, Israel (health ministry), France (French Agency for Food) and the UK (British Dietetic Association). There are over 170 scientific studies that confirm the harmful effects of consuming soy, linking it with infertility, immune system disorders, digestive distress, heart disease, accelerated risk of cancers, thyroid dysfunction, ADD/ADHD, loss of sex drive, lethargy, constipation, weight gain and fatigue.

Soy is also considered one of the top 8 allergens, containing 16–39 allergenic proteins.

Labelling

Check labels and you'll find some form of soy isolate (lecithin or protein) in many processed packaged foods from animal feed to muscle-building protein powders. **It's hidden on labels as:**
Soy protein isolate, soy flour, hydrolyzed vegetable protein, textured vegetable protein, soybean oil, vegetable oil, tofu and lecithin.

Some of the processing soy undergoes produces excitotoxins such as glutamate (like MSG) and aspartate (a component of aspartame), which can cause brain-cell death.

Baby Formula

Because children are developing all the systems and organs of their body, they are highly sensitive to any toxin. Avoid feeding your kids soy formula, as it may harm their developing brains and systems.

SYNTHETIC TRANS FATS

Hydrogenating fats turn plant oils into lifeless oils, removing all of their natural benefits. It increases the shelf life of a product so it can sit in warehouses and supermarket shelves for years before you buy it and eat it.

Hydrogenated fats and oils are new fats created in labs solely for business purposes. Plant-based oils are cheaper than animal fat. The industry decided they could change the molecular structure of vegetable oil so that it would be solid at room temperature, and this way, they could use it instead of butter. This is how they created margarine. Like soy, sold for years as a health food, margarine is the closest thing to plastic. If you put margarine in your garden, no

|55|

insect will come near it, because it's not food. Margarine, a modern fake food, is still used in pastries, baking, cookies and crackers instead of butter because it lasts forever and is much cheaper than butter. The only problem is that every time the industry creates a new fake food substance, we are not told about its effect on our bodies, nor which foods they add it to. Trans fats increase "bad" LDL cholesterol and decrease "good" HDL cholesterol. This is worse than eating only bad cholesterol. All foods that contain trans fats are harmful to our bodies and interfere in natural processes. These fats have been associated with heart disease, breast and colon cancer, atherosclerosis and high cholesterol.

Look out for partially hydrogenated oil, hydrogenated oil, or any fat in all processed and packaged foods as well as in freshly baked pastries (sadly).

ARTIFICIAL FLAVOURS

Believe it or not, most processed foods are artificially flavoured. When food is processed, it loses its fresh flavour. There are over 3,000 different types of artificial flavourings and aromas. These chemicals have been linked to side effects from nervous system depression, dizziness, chest pain, headaches, fatigue, allergies, brain damage, seizures, genetic defects, to tumours and nausea. Yet they are still used in our food.

One artificial flavour can contain many chemicals. For example, strawberry artificial flavouring can contain up to 50 chemical ingredients. When you choose foods next time, even herbal teas, ensure that the aromas and flavours come from a real food, like orange extract rather than orange flavouring.

ARTIFICIAL COLOURS

Any food that comes in a package may contain artificial colouring. Although it doesn't sound too harmful, most of these dyes are made from nasty toxic chemicals which interfere with our brain's and body's functioning. Colour additives have been closely linked to hyperactivity and ADD/ADHD. Artificial colours are found in things like fruit juices and soft drinks, salad dressings, sweets, ready-made foods, meat and now farmed salmon.

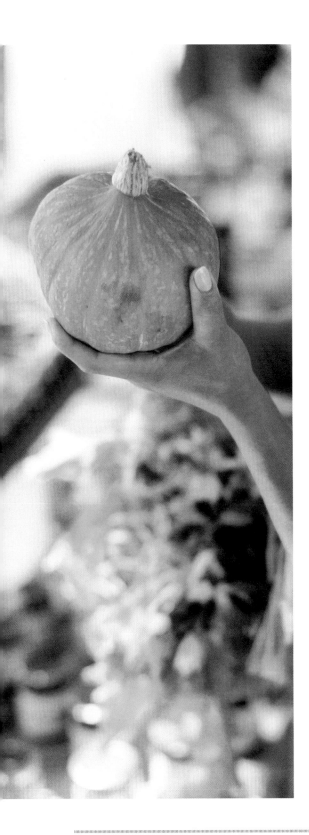

MONOSODIUM GLUTAMATE (MSG)

MSG is a flavour enhancer. From packaged premade sauces, frozen meals and fast foods, to soups, ready-made foods, canned food and junk snacks, MSG has become rather useful in food processing because it stimulates our taste buds and makes any old food taste fresh and delicious. MSG is a neurotoxin that can cause brain cell damage. It's deliberately added to food to help it sell better because it's also addictive. People have experienced side effects ranging from headaches and dizziness to itchy skin, respiratory, digestive and circulatory issues.

IF YOU CAN'T PRONOUNCE IT, DON'T EAT IT

Preservatives make food last longer. There are natural preservatives: putting lemon on avocado, for example, keeps it from going brown. In packaged food, there are always preservatives, unless stated. Preservatives are chemicals that increase convenience but do more harm to the body than good. Start reading labels. Choose foods with the shortest ingredients list, and **if you can't pronounce it, don't eat it.**

FROM HUNTING TO FACTORY SLAUGHTERHOUSES: NATURAL MEAT VS FACTORY FARMED MEAT

Meat is one of the foods most affected by the industrialization of our food supply. We've gone from shepherds and grass-grazing animals to laboratory factories that grow meat for mass production – we're a long way from nature. In the past 50 years, we have gone from eating less than 50 million tons of meat per year to more than 200 million tons globally. The amount of animal waste produced is 130 times more than the amount of human waste. This alone is causing more environmental and health problems than ever before.

Our hunter-gatherer ancestors ate meat sporadically when they made a kill or were celebrating and chose to sacrifice one of their own cattle. Now we expect to eat meat every day, and in many cases at every meal! The monthly village feast has become an every-meal, multi-billion-dollar industry with factories slaughtering thousands of tons of animals per week. Not only is this not a sustainable way of eating, it is damaging the planet, fuelling deforestation and polluting our air.

Did you know that It takes 160 times more land, water and fuel resources to sustain a beef eater's diet than someone on a plant-based diet?

Nowadays we produce enough calories to feed 11 billion people worldwide (more than the human population), yet most of this food is fed to livestock, not hungry people.

The water that's used to raise livestock for food purposes only is more than half the water used in many countries.

The waste from livestock is polluting our planet eight times more than human waste does.

Meat has far less quality today than it did in the past when shepherds cared for cattle, cattle ate grass, absorbed sunlight, and were happy! Not only is the quality of the meat poorer because we have changed these animals' natural diet, but unhappy animals make unhealthy food, because the chemicals that are produced when an animal is unhappy will remain in its meat. In other words, factory farmed meat is less nutritious than it used to be when cows only ate grass.

LIVESTOCK REALITY

How many of us realize that the hamburger or hot dog we have just eaten was a living animal? I think we often forget that we eat of lot of dead animals, and that their quality of life and health obviously plays a role in our bodies when we eat them. So, when it comes to meat, maybe it should be more about quality than quantity. It's no secret how these animals are brought up, slaughtered and prepared for supermarket sale, or is it? The journalist Michael Pollan changed his life when he found that it was illegal to publish photos taken inside a slaughterhouse. What is the big secret? What are they hiding from us? Animals are considered objects for food production and profit, and they are little cared for if not abused and mutilated. This might sound harsh, but this is the reality of what we are doing to our so-called friends. Most slaughterhouses around the world refuse requests for interviews and any attempts to enter these facilities with camera equipment are instantly rejected. Industrial factory-produced meat can no longer be considered a natural whole food or real food. Meat has become the product of a multibillion-dollar business model in which living creatures are involved.

"It's not alright that people can buy a whole chicken for just a few pounds/euros/dollars and not even for a moment think that it was once a living creature. We need to change how our food is produced and move away from cheap industrial food production."

Jenny, a mother of two in Germany

|59|

"If people want to eat meat, they should pay attention to the type of life the animal led and demand quality. When buying designer clothes or cars, people do that, so why is it different with our food?"

Laura, 32, Pilot, Madrid

BUSINESS ONLY WORKS IF PEOPLE BUY THE PRODUCTS.

If food is made to create profit, and we choose what to spend our money on, then we, the consumer, run the market with our food choices.

There's a reason no one knows the effects most of these foods and products have on our lives and planet, because if we knew, we would definitely not be buying them.

Better choices for our bodies and the planet are not more expensive. In fact, it is evident that if thousands of us opted for natural organic food, the price would decrease. It might take longer to get our governments to make smarter investments. Rather than subsidizing corn, wheat and dairy farms they could help reduce the prices of organic foods that are friendlier to our body and planet.

The truth sometimes hurts, and with meat, it definitely hurts! Eating meat is not bad, but industrial factory-farmed meat is not healthy, real food.

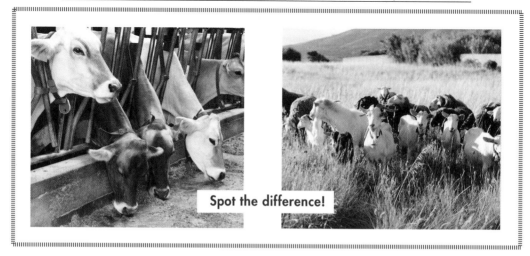

Spot the difference!

WE NEED TO GET FOOD SMART!

The real food dilemma for our generation is how to become a real food wizard. We need to get to the bottom of our food industry and be more conscious of our food choices, so that we're making smarter choices for our bodies, minds and the planet!

SUPERMARKET

Shop at local farmers markets where there is less or no food seduction. Support your local farmers and ask them how they protect their crops from insects. Farmers are great to speak to, and supporting them is fun and better for the planet.

MONTHLY DELIVERY

I avoid supermarkets altogether. Order your staples like grains, beans, nuts, oils, toilet paper and detergents monthly and have them delivered to your home. It saves you time, money and energy!

If you go to the supermarket, avoid the aisles you now know are 100 per cent pure seduction – with all that colourful packaging lighting up your brain chemistry. Head straight for the real food – the fresh vegetables and fruits. Fill your basket and then head to the grains. Now breathe, and do not go near the bakery, confectionery or cereal aisles.

Buy dry grains and beans in bulk. This saves you time and money – bulk is always a better bargain. If possible, order them online and organic.

FOOD CHOICES

Remember that we send messages with every euro, dollar or pound we spend. When we buy natural real foods, we are voting for more of that. When we buy processed products with toxic effects on our body and the planet, we are sending out a message that we don't care. Vote and be heard with what you choose to spend your energy and money on.

Kitchen Organization

Organize your fridge and pantry in a friendly manner so that it suits your new dietary choices. For example:

1. Create a grains cupboard with all your grains stored in airtight glass containers, so it's easy for you to recognize them!

2. Create a snack drawer with trail mixes, almond butter, coconut oil, maple syrup and wheat-free crackers.

3. Create a healthy snack section in the fridge with hummus, pesto, carrots and other easy-to-grab snacks.

4. Organize the fridge so that veggies are prioritized and separated for salads and for cooking, so it's easy to make a meal.

5. Allow your healthier plant-based foods to be easier to access in the fridge, and in the kitchen in general.

6. Buy organic. Check out the organic produce guides "clean fifteen" and "dirty dozen" to prioritize when budgeting (see Chapter 8).

Get Food Smarter:

1. Take the super out of super-market – go to the market.

2. Order your shopping staples online or have them delivered – this saves time, money and energy!

3. Spend that time at home making delicious nutritious meals! Get groovy cooking more often.

4. When you buy packaged foods, like jarred chick-peas, coconut yogurt or granola – read your labels and question where your food comes from.

5. Check out the meal plan ideas (p.268–71) to get a vision of what a week of loving real good food looks like.

SHOPPING TIPS

Use the shopping list on the next three pages to discover a world of veggies, grains, beans and legumes! Veggies and fruits are seasonal so be sure to keep them local. Shopping at farmer's markets will keep your supply local and safe!

Vegetables

acorn squash	lettuce
artichokes	mushrooms (portobello,
asparagus	chestnut, shitake etc.)
beetroots/beets	okra/lady fingers
broccoli	onions
Brussels sprouts	parsley
butternut squash	parsnips
cabbages	peas (frozen)
carrots	peppers
cauliflower	radishes
celery	rocket/arugula
chicory/endives	romaine
collard greens	spinach
coriander	sprouts and baby greens
courgette/zucchini	(if available, such as
cucumber	sunflower, green and pea
garlic	greens)
green beans (all varieties)	sweet potatoes
kale	Swiss chard
kohlrabi	turnips
leeks	watercress

Fruits

Fruit has become less nutritious and sweeter with advanced technology and genetic engineering. They are also harvested earlier and stored longer. I save my tropical fruit feasts for when I'm in Brazil or Hawaii! In Portugal and European countries, I choose local berries, apples and pears. Choose seasonal and local fruits.

avocado	grapes
lemons	berries
tomatoes	bananas
green apples	kiwi fruits
limes	melons (in season)

Fermented Foods

(Choose raw, naturally fermented and unpasteurized options)

sauerkraut   organic miso
kimchi

Natural Sweeteners

maple syrup   dates (medjool)
coconut sugar   raisins
organic raw honey   dried cranberries
stevia leaf   molasses

Nuts and Seeds

*Buy raw and fresh and in bulk, and store in your fridge
or freezer!*

almonds   pine nuts
sunflower seeds   pecans
pumpkin seeds   walnuts
chia seeds   hazelnuts
flaxseeds   almond butter
sesame seeds   tahini (sesame seed paste)
hemp seeds

Gluten-free Grains

quinoa   wild rice
millet   oats/oat flakes
brown rice   (must say gluten free)
red rice   teff
amaranth   rice noodles
buckwheat

Healthy Fats for Cooking and Salad dressing

virgin olive oil   sesame oil
unrefined coconut oil   toasted sesame oil

Flour

(I like to grind my own flour with a high-speed blender)

buckwheat flour
quinoa flour
potato flour

millet flour
oat flour

Beans and Legumes

For sprouting and cooking. If you're just beginning all of this, feel free to buy a few glass-jarred beans and chickpeas to facilitate the process at first. However, buy the dried versions too so you can get sprouting!

mung
adzuki
lentils (all colours)
chickpeas
white

black
pinto
lima
fenugreek seeds for
sprouting!

Fresh Herbs

basil
parsley
coriander
ginger
thyme
rosemary

mint
chives
dill
lemongrass
lime leaves (frozen)
tarragon

Dried Seasonings

Himalayan salt or fleur de
sel
black pepper
turmeric
mustard seeds

paprika
dried thyme
coriander seeds

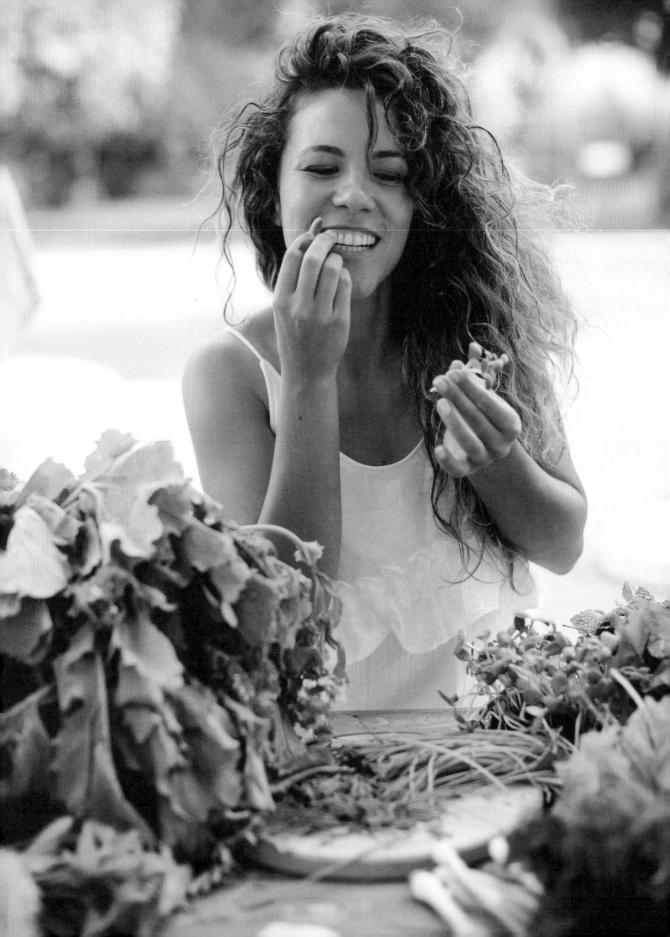

Greens are the only things in the whole world that can make edible energy from sunlight! It's like eating liquid sunshine!

Chapter 3

EAT MORE GREEN LEAVES!

GREEN MEANS GO!

RAW GREEN LEAFY VEGETABLES ARE AN INCREDIBLY CONCENTRATED SOURCE OF NUTRIENTS. THEY CONTAIN EXCEPTIONAL AMOUNTS OF VITAMINS AND MINERALS THAT PROTECT OUR CELLS FROM POLLUTION, TOXINS AND DAMAGE.

Green leaves are completely underrated – at least by humans! Animals know what they're doing. Greens are superfoods, packed with nutrients. That's why so many big, strong animals – from muscular gorillas to enormous elephants – thrive on green leaves! Green leaves are easily accessible and very affordable. They are one of the lowest calorie, lowest sugar foods, and the only way you can get chlorophyll (I'll explain what that is in a bit). In my opinion, **leafy greens are the number one food that we don't have enough of in our modern diet, and this is one of the reasons for so much disease.**

The benefits of greens are endless. They strengthen the blood, immune system and respiratory system – in fact, they are beneficial for every system in our body; their incredible nutrient composition benefits every organ differently.

I like to get my greens in the morning in a juice or smoothie, when my body immediately absorbs all the nutrients and keeps me ahead of the game for the rest of the day.

I'm a huge fan of homemade salad dressing – I won't eat salad without a good dressing, and lots of it! My secret lies in having homemade dressings always stocked in the fridge, ready to use. I believe that any child will devour a salad if the dressing is good! I proved this throughout high school when all my friends licked their plates clean after eating my mum and dad's famous salad dressings.

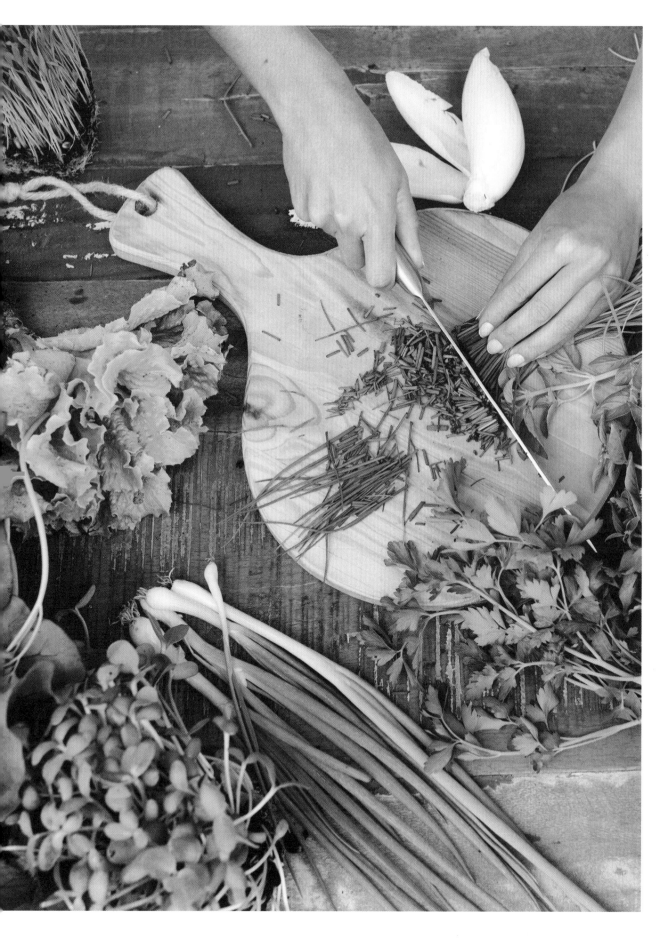

EAT GREENS FIRST

Growing up, for me salad was always the starter at any meal. Super hungry, as kids always are, we gobbled down our salads. My parents didn't make salad a big deal; it was just the norm that you had to eat the salad before the meal was served. This created a healthy habit for each of us (all my siblings love a good salad) and it's a perfect way to crowd out less nutritious foods, without completely removing them from the table. Make your salad colourful and exciting!

WHY ARE GREENS SO GREAT?

Green leaves are the only organisms that can make energy from sunlight! If you eat one thing for your vitality and quality of life, make it green, leafy vegetables. Green leaves transform sunlight into consumable energy. Without green leaves, there is nothing – nothing else would exist. These green leaves are the superfoods of our generation, so, seriously, get your leafy greens in first thing in the morning with a juice or smoothie. Your body will thank you!

ENERGETIC FUNCTION IN THE BODY

In Ayurveda greens have a bitter and astringent taste and create space in the body, so if we are stagnant or clogged up these will help to clear stagnation and dry mucous, and they have anti-inflammatory actions.

Not only are they amazing for our bodies, leafy greens are crucial for our existence on this planet – they make oxygen, purify the air, and therefore promote sustainability. Maybe the world would have more oxygen if we produced more green leaves rather than animals.

In Chinese medicine, green is related to the liver, emotional stability and creativity. It's also the colour of heart energy and supports the functioning of the heart!

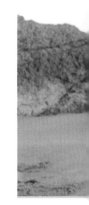

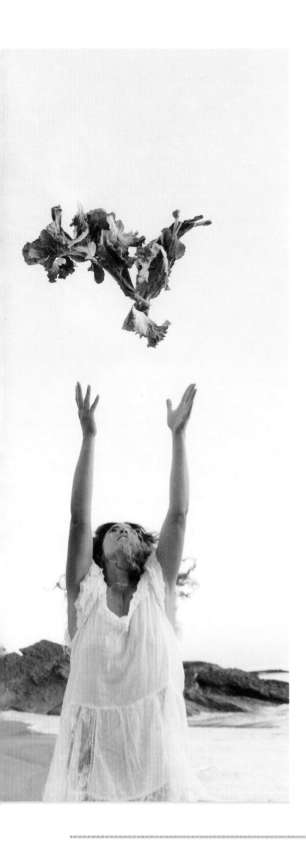

Five Ways to Get Your Dose of Leafy Greens

Leafy greens should occupy the biggest portion on your plate. Here's how to trick yourself into eating them and disguise them in your diet:

1. Juice! Drink your greens first thing in the morning in a juice or smoothie.

2. Throw them into soups and stews just before serving so they are partially raw.

3. Cook your greens with delicious herbs and spices. For example, sauté with garlic and ginger.

4. Stuff 'em into your sandwich (and hide them in your family's sandwiches too!).

5. Serve salad as a starter: at the beginning of a meal, everyone is hungry and will eat what's in front of them. This creates healthy habits for life and is a perfect way to crowd out less nutritious food. AND become a master at dressings. Any child will love a salad that's well dressed!

CHLOROPHYLL

Chlorophyll is the green pigment in green leaves and vegetables. It's what makes green leaves so amazing and helps turn sunlight into food energy through photosynthesis. **Eating chlorophyll is like eating liquid sunshine** (how exciting is that?). It's the first product of light. Researchers say that it contains more healing properties than any other substance. All life on this planet comes from the sun. Only green plants can transform the sun's energy into food!

Chlorophyll is the "life-blood" of plants, and its molecular structure is almost identical to that of our human blood cells. The only difference between chlorophyll and red blood cells is the centre that holds each cell together. In red blood cells, it's iron, and in chlorophyll (plant "blood" cells), it's magnesium. Because they're so similar, chlorophyll helps our blood deliver oxygen around the body. So, yes, when we drink green juice or eat lots of leafy greens, we could say that we are drinking the highest concentration of liquid sunshine and life blood!

During World War I, when the medics ran out of blood plasma on the battlefield, doctors used transfusions of chlorophyll instead.

Greens are a source of:

* calcium
* magnesium
* iron
* potassium
* phosphorous
* zinc
* vitamins A, C, E and K
* fibre
* folic acid
* micronutrients
* phytochemicals

Where do you think the calcium in cow's milk comes from? It's the grass, not the milk! Cows don't make calcium, so it can only be from the food they eat. If cows are not fed grass, their milk is not rich in calcium because they are not getting their leafy greens!

Benefits of eating greens:

* Blood purification – it's almost like we get a blood transfusion each time we eat a salad
* Cancer prevention
* Improved circulation

|72|

* Strengthened immune system
* Healthy intestinal flora
* Subtle, light and flexible energy
* A lifted spirit and less depression
* Improved liver, gallbladder and kidney function
* Cleared congestion, especially in lungs by a reduction of mucus
* Increased alkalinity

There are a wide variety of greens available year-round, so explore options that you can enjoy locally. If you get bored with your favorites, be adventurous and experiment with new greens that you've never tried before. Some leafy greens have little flavour, such as spinach, lettuce and kale, so they're easy to disguise in smoothies, juices and sandwiches. Some give flavour, such as rocket and parsley, while others are even spicy, such as watercress and chives. Be adventurous and experiment.

The adjacent list shows some of the most nutritious leafy greens for you to choose from. Try and pick a different one each day.

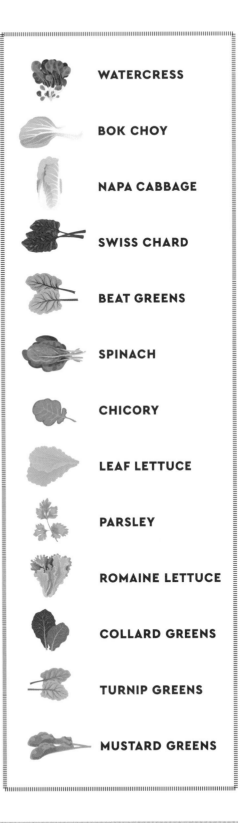

WATERCRESS

BOK CHOY

NAPA CABBAGE

SWISS CHARD

BEAT GREENS

SPINACH

CHICORY

LEAF LETTUCE

PARSLEY

ROMAINE LETTUCE

COLLARD GREENS

TURNIP GREENS

MUSTARD GREENS

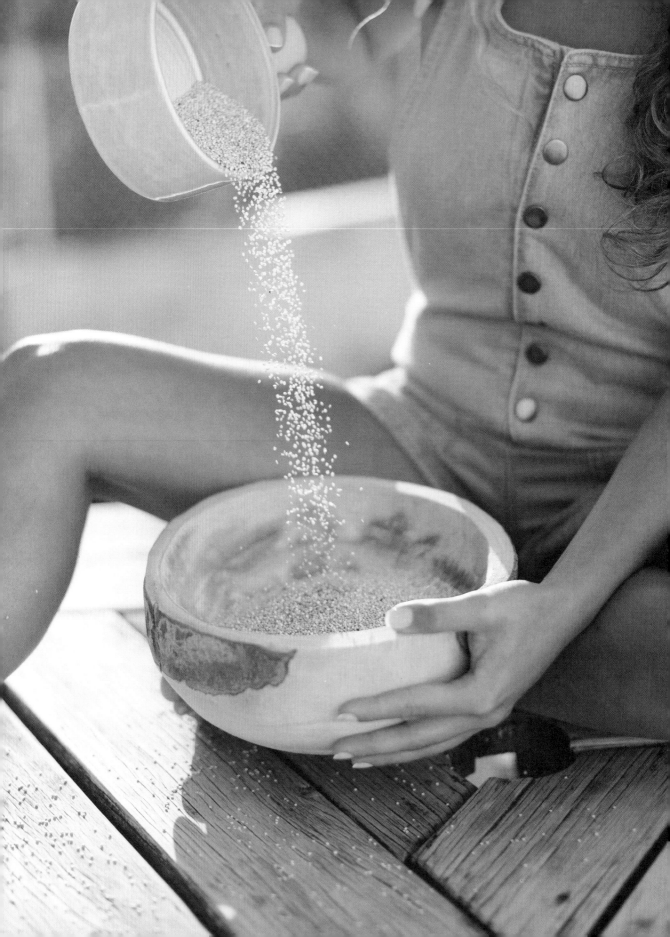

Whole grains are grounding foods. They connect us to the earth and help us feel more focused, stable and grounded in life.

Chapter 4

STOCK UP ON WHOLY GRAINS

SUSTAIN WITH GRAINS

TRADITIONAL CULTURES SEE WHOLE GRAINS AS GROUNDING, CONNECTING US TO THE EARTH AND HELPING US BE MORE FOCUSED – LITERALLY MAKING US FEEL MORE STABLE AND GROUNDED IN LIFE.

I used to avoid grains as a teenager. I thought they made me fat. It wasn't until I started travelling around the world and eating with different cultures that I learned how important grains are to human existence and vitality. And how delicious they are! Did you know that grains are one of the few natural whole foods with a very long shelf life? These miracle foods offer abundant amounts of energy, protein, fibre, vitamins and minerals, and used to be extremely important when fresh fruits and veggies were scarce.

Grains have sustained civilizations for thousands of years. Each region of the world has its native grain, which we can see in traditional dishes: corn (the Americas), quinoa and amaranth (Peru, Mexico), wholegrain rice (Asia), sorghum (Africa), teff (Ethiopia), wheat (Middle East), burghul and couscous (Europe), and buckwheat (Russia).

My favourite grain is quinoa. The Incas thrived on this grain for centuries. With high protein levels, quinoa is a perfect grain to get into your kitchen. Easy, quick and versatile! It only takes 20 minutes to cook, and you can enjoy it salty or sweet.

Whole grains are rich sources of:
* *iron*
* *magnesium*
* *vitamin E*
* *B-complex vitamins*
* *phytochemicals*
* *antioxidants*
* *fibre*
* *protein*

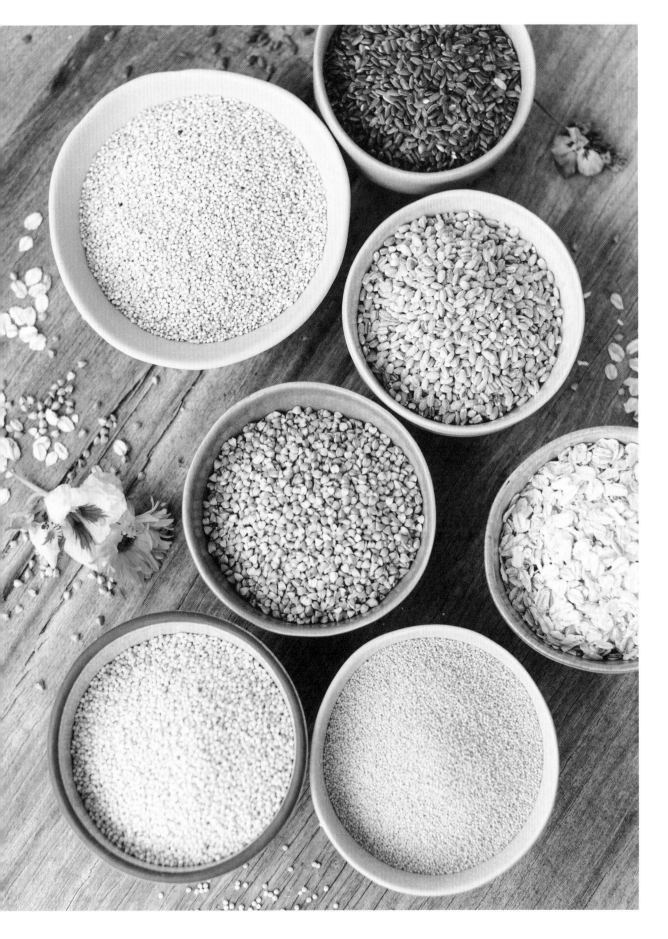

NO-LONGER WHOLY GRAINS

Whole grains are seeds packed with nutrients and energy so that they can grow to become bigger plants. In nature, a grain grows with a skin or shell that protects it and provides proteins and nutrients so that it can grow. Since the industrialization of food, we throw away the shell and germ (with all the nutrients) and only eat the sugary part in the middle. The modern food industry basically produces foods from grains that have been peeled of essential nutrients, protein and fibre. Nowadays, we are only eating the calories of the grain – and no nutrition. Personally, if I'm going to eat sugar, I'd rather eat chocolate cake – once in a while – than nutrient-less grains.

White bread, white flour, pasta, breakfast cereals, biscuits, crackers, pizza dough, pastries, cookies and cake are all made of refined, processed and chemically bleached grains.

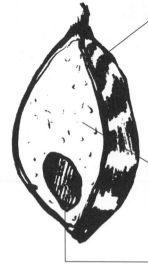

BRAN
fibre and protein-rich outer protective layer.

ENDOSPERM
carbohydrate inner core.

GERM
vitamins, minerals, essential healthy fats and antioxidants.

WHAT'S THE DIFFERENCE?

Rice with its husk is packed with nutrition, but rice without its shell is empty calories.

A grain is made up of the bran, endosperm and germ. When grains are refined the bran and germ are removed. All that's left over is the sugary inner core. Refined wheat, for example, is then used to make white bread and other white flour products. This process is done for industrial reasons and not for our health.

The bran is the fibre-rich outer layer that protects the seed and contains protein, fibre, B vitamins and trace minerals.

The endosperm is the middle core that contains carbohydrates (sugars) which provide energy for the seed to sprout to form a plant.

The germ is the part of the seed that actually sprouts! It is very nutrient rich and contains antioxidants, vitamin E, B vitamins, minerals and healthy fats. We definitely want to be eating the bran and germ!

BE NOT FOOLED

When you buy foods made of grains that make positive health claims, like cereals and bread, check the labels for 100 per cent whole grains. If the package says "whole grains" or "rich in fibre", it can simply be good marketing and the product might actually contain a majority of refined grains. So, check labels for 100 per cent whole grain flour.

A LITTLE ON FIBRE

My superhero! Fibre is an essential nutrient missing from many modern diets today – one reason being that we are removing it from all our grains for no good reason. It's mostly found in plant foods and its benefits are never ending. Fibre is not absorbed into the body. It travels through the digestive tract, acting like a sponge, soaking up and sweeping out toxins, "bad" cholesterol and heavy metals, among other unwanted substances. Without fibre, we are not cleaning out our intestines and therefore reabsorbing a lot of waste. Eek! Fibre also feeds the good bacteria in our guts (prebiotic).

I'm sure you've heard people refer to soluble and insoluble fibre. The main difference between these is that soluble fibre absorbs water and creates a sort of gel-like substance in your intestines, which pulls toxins, cholesterol and other impurities out of the gut. Insoluble fibre creates bulk which helps to move the stool along more quickly and keeps you regular.

Benefits of eating fibre:

* *Increases satiety*
* *Zero calories*
* *Cleanses the intestinal wall*
* *Removes toxins*
* *Reduces cholesterol*
* *Reduces caloric absorption*
* *Regulates blood sugar levels*
* *Keeps us fuller for longer*
* *Improves intestinal health*
* *Regulates bowel movements*
* *Feeds your good bacteria!*

CHOOSING OUR GRAINS

There are so many more grains beyond white rice, white flour (wheat), rye and spelt. There are a number of delicious ancient grains that sustained our ancestors. Check out my favourite seven whole grains.

These **seven sexy grains are all gluten-free**, super easy to cook and versatile. You can enjoy 'em savoury or sweet, for breakfast, lunch, dinner or dessert!

Gluten can be a problem for many people, which is why I have excluded it here, and why my favourite grains are naturally gluten-free! More on this in Chapter 8: Cut The Crap.

* quinoa
* millet
* red rice
* brown rice
* buckwheat
* amaranth
* teff

The only way to get the holy from grains is to cook and eat them WHOLE. Put some music on and get groovy in the kitchen; experiment and find out what you like best.

How to cook grains:

* *One cup of grains (dry) yields enough for two to four people*
* *Always wash grains before cooking, especially quinoa – quinoa has a natural "pesticide", saponin, that protects it from being eaten by birds and insects. Saponin washes off with water!*
* *See the table overleaf for grain-to-water ratio*
* *Cooking length can depend on the heat of a stove (see table overleaf for cooking times)*
* *Toward the end of the cooking time, lift the lid and check if there's enough water to prevent burning the grains. (I prefer my grains fluffy so I add more water than necessary to prevent burning and remove the lid toward the end so excess water can evaporate)*
* *Do not stir your grains, unless you're making risotto!*
* *Taste to check if they are fully cooked*

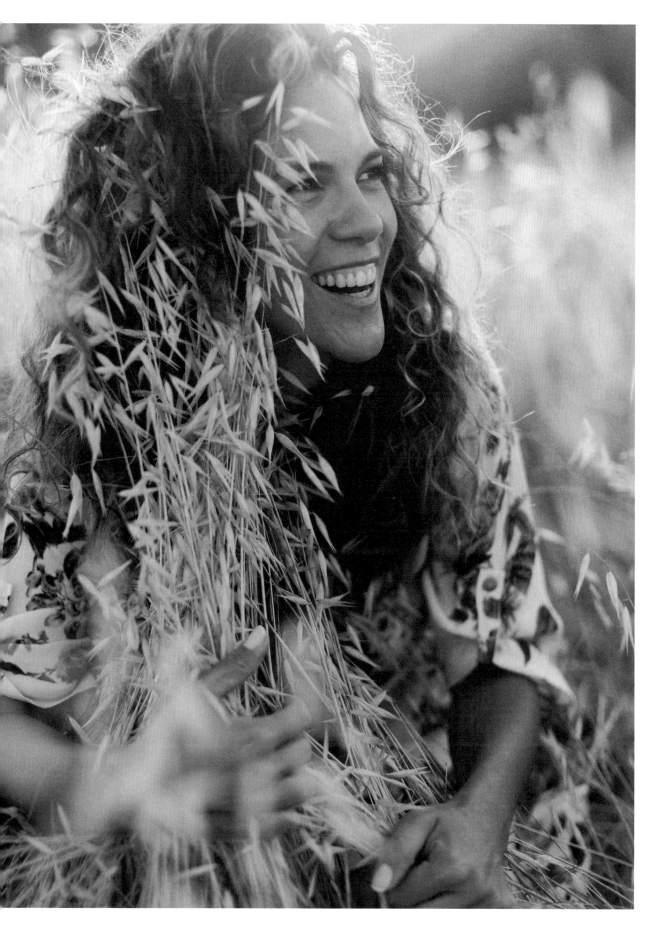

COOK ONCE, EAT THREE TIMES

Since cooked grains keep very well in the fridge, you can always cook more than you need and have the leftovers the next day. For example, cook a batch of quinoa at night, have it with your dinner, refrigerate the rest, and have it in the morning as porridge; have the third portion accompanying a salad for lunch. It's really convenient. I do this all the time and it makes meal planning so much easier!

Five Ways To Get More Grains Into Your Diet

1. Turn to the shopping lists in Chapter 2: Love Real Food (p.63–5) and buy these great grains! While you're at it, buy eight air-tight glass containers to store these pretty grains and make some space in your kitchen. Some are best used as flour, like buckwheat, while others are perfect as a whole grain!

2. Now that they're in your kitchen, treat them just like rice, make a risotto, or add caramelized onions, garlic and spices for an instantly delicious dish to have with your normal meal.

3. Get groovy by grinding these grains into flour and making your homemade pancakes, cakes, muffins and bread! Buckwheat flour, rice flour and teff flour are perfect replacements for wheat flour.

4. Stuff them into veggies such as peppers and courgettes.

5. Enjoy granola or a warming porridge as a snack.

Yum! Enjoy these great grains!

COOKING GRAINS

1 CUP OF GRAIN		WATER	COOKING TIME	CONTAINS GLUTEN?
FAVOURITE 7 GRAINS (ALL GLUTEN-FREE)	Quinoa	2.2 cups	15–20 mins	no
	Millet	2 cups	30 mins	no
	Brown/ red rice	2 cups	30 mins	no
	Buckwheat (aka Kasha)	2 cups	20–30 mins	no
	Amaranth	3 cups	30 mins	no
	Teff	4 cups	15–20 mins	no
Oats (whole groats)		3 cups	75–90 mins	buy oats that are labelled as gluten-free
Oatmeal (rolled oats)		2 cups	75–90 mins	questionable due to content, contact, or contamination
Barley (pearled)		2–3 cups	60 mins	yes
Bulgur (cracked wheat)		2 cups	20 mins	yes
Cornmeal (aka Polenta)		3 cups	20 mins	no
Kamut		3 cups	90 mins	yes
Rye berries		3 cups	2 hours	yes
Spelt		3 cups	2 hours	yes
Wheat berries		3 cups	60 mins	no
Wild rice		4 cups	60 mins	no

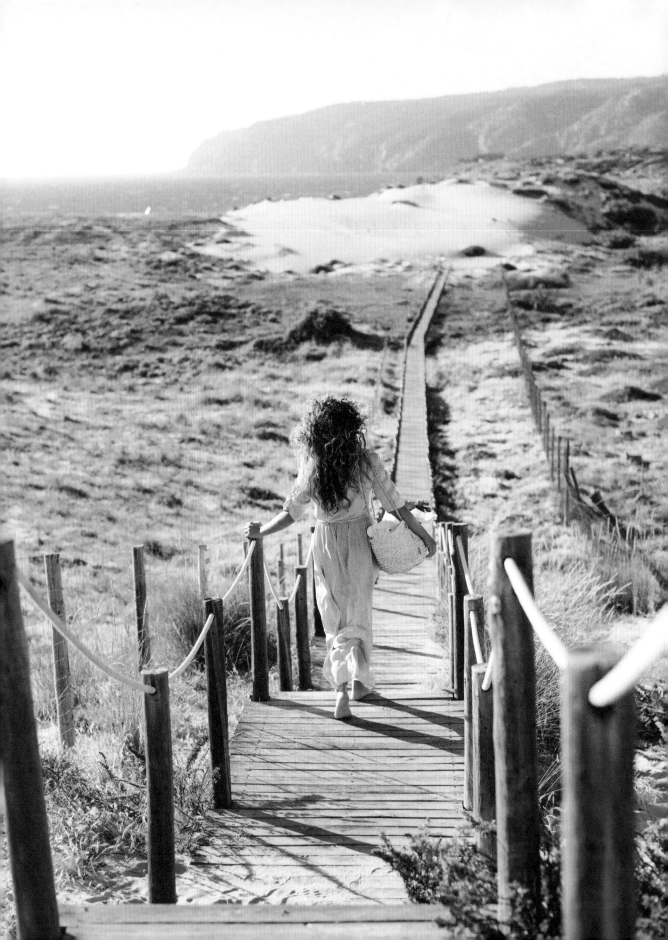

> *"It is in your moments of decision that your destiny is shaped."*
> Anthony Robbins

Chapter 5

DEMYSTIFYING PROTEIN

MAKE AN INFORMED CHOICE

PROTEIN IS ONE OF THE BIGGEST CONTROVERSIES WHEN IT COMES TO NUTRITION. MOST PEOPLE ASSOCIATE PROTEIN WITH ANIMAL PRODUCTS. THIS CHAPTER DEMYSTIFIES PROTEIN AND GIVES YOU THE TOOLS YOU NEED TO MAKE YOUR OWN CHOICES.

MY JOURNEY WITH PROTEIN WAS ONE OF SELF-DISCOVERY AND EXPERIMENTATION. I'M INVITING YOU TO DO THE SAME. STOP LISTENING TO MARKETING PUNS AND SCIENTIFIC STUDIES BACKED AND PAID FOR BY INTEREST GROUPS.

No one knows your body better than you. There is no one right answer, nor do you have to stay committed to one type of protein source for life. Where you live, what you do, what naturally grows around you and what's available to you will influence the needs of your body and what you choose to eat. So, again, we are all unique with individual needs and it's time for us to make the best choices for us. And, of course, our planet.

Understanding the effect our food choices have on the planet may inspire new choices. When it comes to protein, it's a big conversation, often an emotional topic and with much contradicting information. My aim is to demystify the confusion and give you confidence so we can make smarter food choices as a global community.

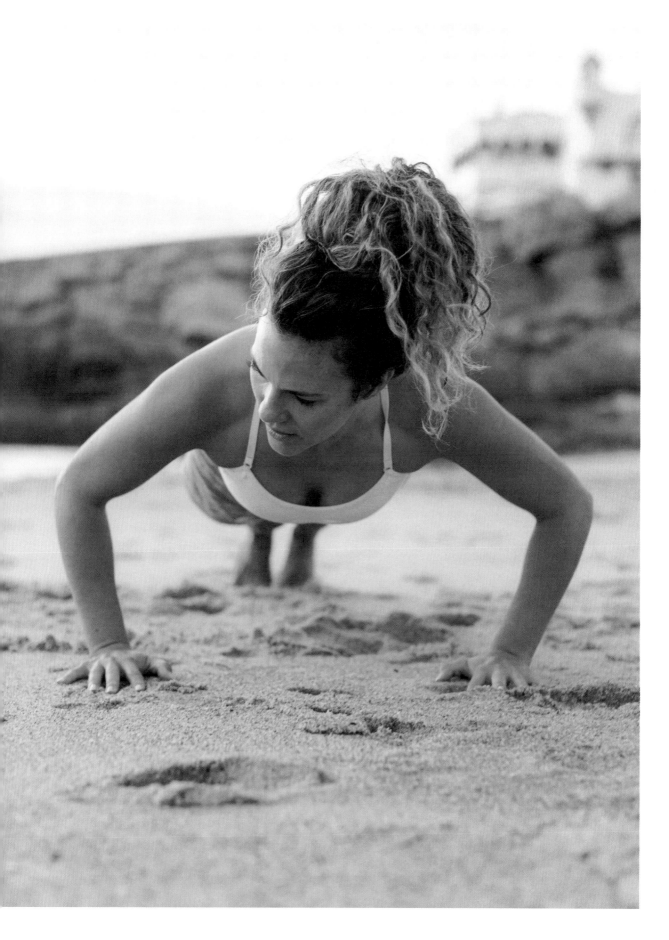

LET'S STICK TO THE FACTS

Protein exists everywhere. Just like our bodies need protein, so do all living animals and plants. So, when we eat plants, vegetables, grains, nuts, seeds, beans, sprouts, land or ocean animals we are always getting protein, always.

First of all, let's look at the basics.

WHAT IS A PROTEIN?

Amino Acids 101: Proteins are the building blocks of the body. They build everything from hormones and enzymes, to muscle, brain and blood cells – every cell in your body is made up of protein. It is used to build, maintain and repair all cell structures – thus the hype of how essential protein is to our diet!

The building blocks of protein are amino acids. There are 22 amino acids, 9 of which are essential – "essential" meaning we have to get them through our diet because our bodies **do not** produce them.

When a food has all 9 essential amino acids, it's considered a "complete" protein food.

PROTEIN SOURCES

Proteins are present in all food that comes from nature. Every food has a different concentration of protein. We can measure protein by 100g or by 100kcal.

Land and ocean animals and their derivatives (dairy and eggs) contain all the nine essential amino acids, and are therefore complete proteins. Nonetheless, vegetables, grains, beans, nuts and seeds are excellent sources of protein too. In fact, there are many benefits to getting our protein from plant-based sources, as they have higher nutrient levels and zero "bad" saturated fat.

Interestingly, vegetables, grains, beans, nuts and seeds have **more protein per calorie than meat.** The myth that protein is not present in plants is because most plant-based forms of protein are missing one or two of the nine essential amino acids, and are therefore "incomplete" proteins. However, once you combine different foods, like vegetables and grains, or grains and beans, it's easy to get all the essential amino acids you need.

I love coming across traditional

cultures that still have a diet based on rice and beans or dhal (lentils). From Brazil to India, this is the case. As a world community, we've thrived on high-energy, protein-rich foods all year round – mainly grains, beans and seasonal vegetables, with occasional hunting. My dad's favourite meal is still rice and beans!

Sources of plant-based protein:
grains, nuts and legumes; wheatgrass; sprouts; chlorella and spirulina; green leafy vegetables; all other vegetables.

Sources of animal protein:
meat (land or water animals); eggs; milk, cheese.

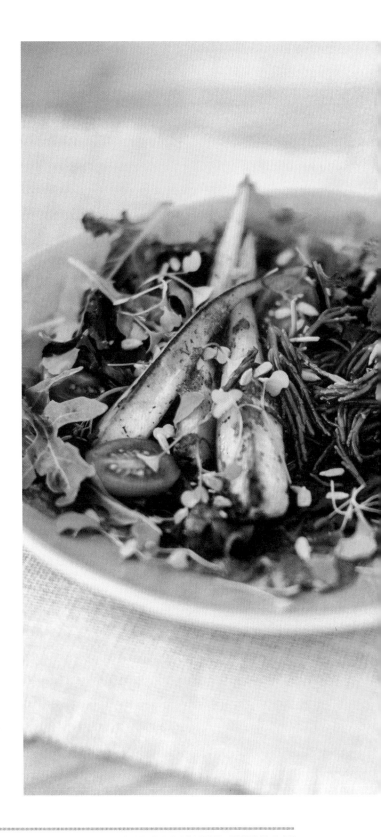

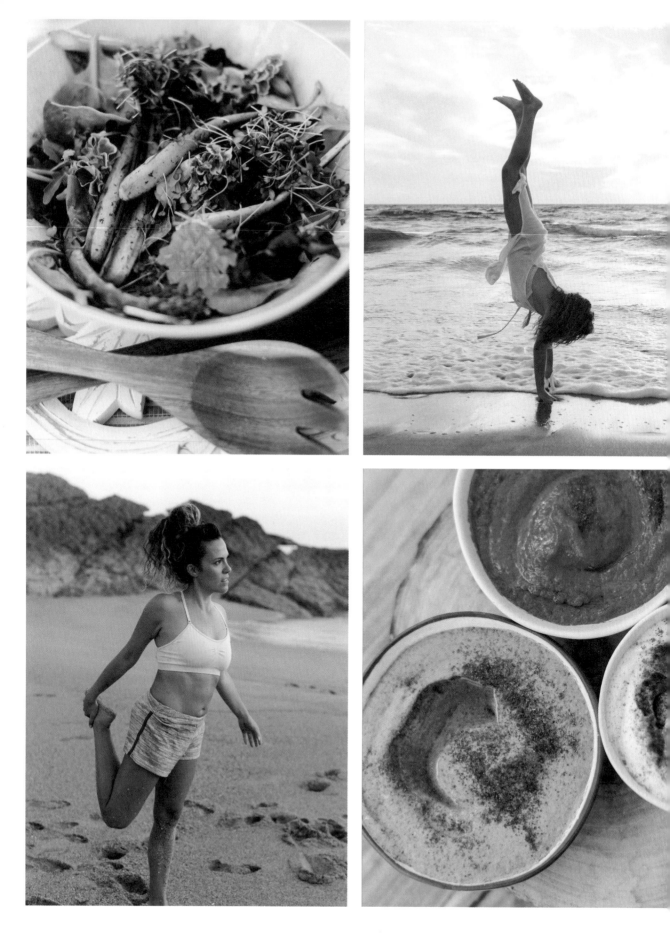

PROTEIN PER 100G

Food	Protein
Potato	2.5g
Spinach	2.9g
Cow Milk (1% fat)	3.4g
Green Peas	5.4g
Brown Rice	7.9g
Macadamia Nuts	7.9g
Tofu	8g
Wheat Bread	13g
Eggs (chicken)	13g
Quinoa	14.1g
Walnuts	15g
Hazelnuts	15g
Chia Seeds	16g
Oats	17g
Cod	17.8g
Cashew Nuts	18g
Flaxseed	18g
Chickpeas	19g
Pumpkin Seeds	19g
Pistachio Nuts	20g
Sirloin Steak	20.3g
Almonds	21g
Pinto Beans	21.4g
Lima Beans	21.5g
Kidney Beans	22.5g
Chicken Breast	23.1g
Tuna Steak	23.4g
Mung Bean Sprouts	24g
Peanut Butter	25g
Lentils	25.8g
Soybeans	36g
Hemp Seed	36.7g
Spirulina Seaweed	57g
Chlorella	58g

How much protein do we need?

Protein recommendations per day for women and men:
Women: 46g
Men: 56g

Formula:

Average protein intake for normal adult – 0.8g protein per kg (according to US Food and Nutrition Board)

Average intake for bodybuilder – Between 1.2 and 1.4g per kg (according to American College of Sports Medicine)

The world's highest source of complete protein: spirulina and blue-green algae

Spirulina is the world's highest source of complete protein (65 per cent protein), as well as being a super source of minerals, trace elements, phytonutrients and enzymes.

PROTEIN MYTHS, DEMYSTIFIED

* *Plant-based protein is easier to absorb by our bodies than the protein in animal products.*
* *Plant-based diets can help prevent over 60 per cent of deaths that are due to chronic disease.*
* *People who pursue a vegetarian diet live longer than meat eaters and have lower rates of death from heart disease.*
* *It IS possible to be healthy and get all the complete protein you need on a plant-based diet with a good variety of grains, vegetables, nuts, seeds and beans.*

* *Many vegetables, including green vegetables, sprouts and beans, have more protein per calorie than meat.*
* *Plant protein-rich foods are also the richest in micronutrients, vitamins, minerals, fibre, bioflavonoids, antioxidants and other phytochemicals.*
* *All plant-based foods in nature contain protein.*
* *By eating more of these high-nutrient, low-calorie, plant-protein foods, our body receives all the protein it needs AND is flooded with protective micronutrients.*

* Animal protein does not contain antioxidants or phytonutrients and can be high in saturated fat, the fat we don't want to eat too much of.
* Gorillas and elephants thrive on only green plants and are massive, muscular animals.
* Protein does not produce muscle; weight-lifting does.

Now that we understand that our food industry is not necessarily created with our vitality in mind and that the animal meat industry is worth billions, it might be time to start connecting the dots and creating our very own experiences. Studies and research have to be funded. When we listen to studies and facts about what foods we should eat, we need to be smarter and ask questions. Who funded the study? If a study declaring coffee to be essential for vitality is funded by the coffee bean company, how credible is that study? The same goes for our meat industry.

Rafael's Story

"I have always been interested in sports and always wanted a muscular body. At sixteen I started to go to the gym, and during the next three years I followed the traditional diet of chicken breast and eggs. I always thought it was necessary because it was what I saw others do. However, as I have always been interested in nutrition, I researched more and more until I discovered that factory-farmed animal protein is not only not necessary, it is even harmful to your health, animals and the planet. Since then, I have adopted a plant-based diet and the results are getting better every day. I have more energy to train and recover faster. If anyone ever tells you that you need animal protein, do not believe them! Eating meat is not a sign of strength or masculinity. Consciousness and taking responsibility for our actions is!"

- Rafael Pinto, age 20, law student and body-builder, Portugal

THE TRUTH ABOUT PLANT-BASED PROTEIN

Many people have the opinion that our bodies need more protein than is normally recommended, and that animal protein is a higher-quality protein than plant-based protein. However, a properly structured plant-based diet is definitely not linked with protein deficiency. In fact, **many studies have shown that a well-planned plant-based diet is powerful in strengthening the body, flushing it with nutrients, preventing and even reversing a host of diseases common in our current era.**

THE TRUTH ABOUT MEAT

The idea that meat is necessary for good health and vitality has been hammered into us repeatedly. And this is even in a time when scientific studies have proven the nutritional benefits of a plant-based diet.

I am not here to convince anyone to be a vegetarian! Rather I would hope to give you the courage to truly understand the effects each of our food choices has on our very own body and on the planet so we can make more sustainable choices.

I feel as though most of us don't realize we are eating animals or their derivatives in almost every snack or meal. Most of us don't know how these animals are fed, raised, "cared" for, or slaughtered. And if we start to think about it, it might be this way for a reason. It is officially prohibited to publish any photos taken inside of a slaughterhouse because of the obvious negative effect it would have on sales.

When did we become obsessive meat eaters? If our ancestors ever ate meat, it was wild meat that they hunted themselves. It was healthy meat with very little fat, and the environment the animal lived in was also healthy. They ate the organs, the bone marrow and boiled the bones for broth. But most of the time, they ate mainly vegetables and grains.

"Humans have no known anatomical, physiological, or genetic adaptations to meat consumption. Quite the opposite, we have many adaptations to plant consumption."
Archeological geneticist, Christina Warriner

Carnivores can make their own vitamin C. If you don't eat plants, you have to make your own vitamin C, so lions make vitamin C, but we don't.

We have a longer digestive tract than carnivores because food needs to stay in our body longer to digest and absorb plant nutrients. Carnivores have very short digestive tracts. Meat putrefies much faster than plants. Our long digestive tract holds meat in for so long that it rots in our intestines!

Land and ocean animals are all wild by nature. Many of us don't realize that all animals have a place in the natural ecosystem that outweighs their value as food. This means that every animal on this planet has a job that no other animal can do. When we start to interfere with the natural diversity and existence of different animals, especially wild ones, we are putting our own ecosystem and existence in danger.

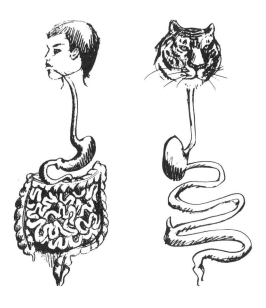

Human vs carnivore digestive system.

REASONS TO REDUCE OR AVOID EATING ANIMAL PROTEIN

Most of our meat is now mass produced, a process that is toxic to our food and our environment. It's rare to find naturally farmed animal meat and animal products.
Did you know that many beach restaurants sell farmed fish? Next time you should ask and see.

If proteins are essentially amino acids, overeating them will cause acidity in the body. Animal foods are considered inflammatory, acid-forming foods. More reasons to avoid these foods include:

* Genetic engineering
* Low nutrient content. Most meat doesn't beat iceberg lettuce for nutritional value
* Bovine growth hormone
* Cow disease
* Poor quality
* Difficult to digest
* Parasites
* Intestinal health
* Risk of disease and cancer

* **Heart disease.** *Dr Dean Ornish and Dr Caldwell Esselstyn have continuously proven through their patients that the absence of meat can reverse heart disease.*
* **Food-borne illness.** *Several governmental bodies state that chicken and other meats are sources of food-borne illnesses despite the heavy use of pesticides and antibiotics.*
* **Nitrites in processed meat (like hot dogs, sausages and ham) are associated with the two leading childhood cancers – brain tumours and childhood leukemia.** *Hot dogs have some of the highest levels!*
* **Factory-farmed animals contain toxic chemicals.** *Meat accumulates pesticides and toxic chemicals up to 14 times more than in plant foods.*
* **Antibiotics.** *Corn-fed beef becomes acidic and more susceptible to disease. Today, cows are fed low doses of antibiotics in their corn feed to help combat their low immunity and acidic bodies.*

|96|

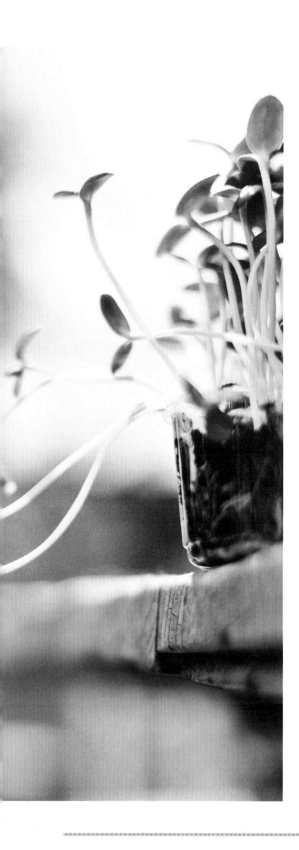

* **The top fifteen foods that cause advanced glycation (aging) all come from animals.**
* *An acid naturally found in animal foods (arachidonic acid) is linked to brain inflammation, depression, anxiety and stress.*
* *Both land- and ocean-farmed animals no longer eat their natural diet. Natural plant eaters like fish and cows are being fed animal remains such as ground organs and leftovers, making them unhealthy and sick.*
* *The digestion of all animal products produces acids. This creates acidity throughout the body and blood, which hinders the efficiency of enzymes and vitamins, and even the absorption of nutrients. The harder your body has to work to maintain its mildly alkaline pH the more stress it causes on your body.*
* *Unhealthy animals make unhealthy food.*
* *Overfed and overmedicated animals absorb, store and accumulate toxins at extremely high rates. Most of these toxins are fat-soluble, like dioxins from industrial processes. We absorb these toxins by eating animal products.*
* *Even when meat says "grass fed", there is no regulating body for this. So the animal could have been grass fed just once a month.*

|97|

REASONS TO REDUCE OR AVOID EATING FISH AND SHELLFISH MEAT

* Fish absorb high levels of industrial toxins and heavy metals, and can contain parasites.
* Farmed fish are greatly susceptible to disease and malformation, and are still sold as being edible.
* Farmed fish are fed high levels of antibiotics and foods which are not natural to their species, such as pig and poultry feces (that's right! Eek!), GMO soy and herbicides.
* Intense overcrowding is the norm in fish farms, meaning the fish do not have enough room to swim, which causes sores, sea lice and over-fattening, increasing their ability to absorb toxins.
* Overcrowded fish farms are infested with sea lice, which requires the spraying of pesticides into our oceans and onto our fish.

Farmed salmon, for example, is sprayed with pesticides to prevent sea-lice infestation. These pesticides are now flowing in our sea water!
* Fish and other seafood absorb extremely high levels of chemicals such as arsenic, mercury, PCBs, DDT, dioxins and lead, which are stored in their flesh and fat. They are susceptible to all toxins present in the oceans, which range from pollutants, like sewage, oil spills, to heavy metals and nuclear runoff from power plant leaks.
* Farmed fish, bottom dwellers, eel, shrimp, and other large fish such as tuna harbour higher levels of mercury and toxins due to living at the bottom of the oceans where toxic waste ends up. They are also predators, meaning they accumulate toxins from all the fish they eat, which then ends up in us!
* Wild fish, although they eat their natural diet of plankton and sea algae, are usually not fished sustainably. It's healthier for us, but still not healthy for the planet. Nonetheless, wild fish, especially the larger ones, are still susceptible to being toxic due to the ocean's accumulated toxicity – containing plastic, dioxins, PCBs, pharmaceuticals and so on.
* Line-caught fish is the best

(once in a while) – or go fishing yourself!

ANIMAL WELFARE

* *Inhumane treatment. Animals in factory farms are over-crowded to the point they cannot turn around or spread a wing!*
* *Fish farms crowd thousands of fish into tiny compartments where they end up absorbing their own faeces.*
* *Both land- and ocean-farmed animals are treated like objects and machines – they are pumped with drugs, fed their own waste, and forced to grow and produce as fast as possible, often subjected to twenty-four-hour artificial lighting.*
* *Animals put on weight faster if you don't let them move, so they are kept in small confinements and fed lots of corn and high-carb foods (making them unhealthy).*
* *Fish feel pain. When they are pulled up in nets with tons of fish, many are killed by the weight of the others.*

IF OUR SURVIVAL DEPENDS ON IT... SUSTAINABILITY

Our consumption of animals (involving raising and eating livestock, and harvesting fish) is the single largest contributing factor to the global depletion of natural resources.

* *Reducing animal agriculture is thought to be the most effective way to reduce all environmental issues.*
* *Factory farming is an inefficient use of land, water and energy.*
* *Depletion and over-use of fresh water: it takes 160 times more land, water and fuel resources to sustain a beef eater's diet than a plant-based diet. In order to produce animal products, land, water and energy is required to grow, harvest and transport the feed that is then fed to the farmed animals. We currently produce enough calories to feed 11 billion people worldwide, however, most of this food goes to feed livestock, not hungry people. Once their feed is produced, even more land, water and energy are needed to raise and house the animals, not to mention dispose of their waste, which causes eight times the amount of pollution than human waste. Finally, more energy is required to transport the animals to be slaughtered and process their bodies.*
* *40 per cent of greenhouse gasses are the result of livestock and dairy production.*

The world's cattle alone consume a quantity of food equal to the caloric needs of 8.7 billion people – more than the entire human population on Earth. There are millions of people worldwide that suffer from chronic hunger. Instead of feeding these grains to livestock, feed them to people!

INEFFICIENT USE OF AGRICULTURE

America uses 227 thousand km² (56 million acres) of land for animal agriculture while dedicating only 16 thousand km² (four million acres) to growing produce.

INEFFICIENT USE OF WATER

It takes 1,320 gallons/5 million litres of water to produce a 250g beef steak! You wasted five million litres of water so that you could have your steak last night! The water used to raise animals for food each year is more than half the water used by many countries.

ENVIRONMENTAL POLLUTION

Factory farm animal waste does not fertilize land because the animals aren't healthy. This waste pollutes the ground and ground water. Raising animals for food is the biggest polluter of our water and topsoil.

DESTRUCTION OF NATURAL HABITATS

It takes more land to raise animals for food than plants, to produce the equivalent nutritional value. Rainforests are being destroyed to create room for factory farms, in Brazil, South America and other precious forests around the world. **By choosing to eat more plant-based foods, we can significantly reduce our carbon footprint, save precious water supplies, and help ensure that nutrient-dense crops are fed to people, rather than to livestock.**

"LEAVE US FISH ALONE."

I've never been much of a meat eater, but having grown up by the coast in Portugal, I've always been proud of living where the best-tasting fish can be found. I share everyone's confusion and disappointment in what our industrial world has done to food, especially when it comes to fish. Did you know that oceans produce 50 per cent of the planet's oxygen and absorb greenhouse gasses? That means that without them, we would have no air to breathe.

If I told you that oceans and marine life are being killed, coral reefs are dying, and that it has been estimated that by 2048 we will lose all forms of sea life due to ocean acidification, would you believe me? None of this is due to pollution or climate change. It's due to overfishing. With the rise in demand for fish consumption, no one fishes with a fishing rod anymore.

These are the new common methods of industrial fishing: (WARNING: this may change the way you feel about eating industrialized fish.)

Bottom trawlers – curtain-like nets dropped 30cm into the sandy seafloor and pulled across the seafloor to catch anything that could be sold as fish. Imagine how these destroy coral and kill non-target animals like dolphins, whales, turtles, and other organisms that are vital to marine habitats. This method creates black holes in our oceans that will take thousands of years to grow back – not weeks or months.

Dredging – metal scoops drag along the ocean floor to pick up clams, disturbing all ocean floor life, disturbing the water quality, depleting the ocean floor of oxygen, and making it uninhabitable.

Long hook lines – a practice employed in the open oceans with thousands of baited hooks that are dropped in the water and connected by one long line. This method is unspecific, again catching non-target animals, which are badly injured or killed (fish, turtles, birds, dolphins, whales and other mammals).

Massive seine nets or gillnets – nets that are staked into the ocean floor and dragged, pulling all ocean life with them. These methods are responsible for a staggering amount of bycatch in the past twenty years that amounted to 300,000 dolphins, whales and other mammals, 85,000 sea turtles, 160,000 albatross birds and 3,000,000 sharks.

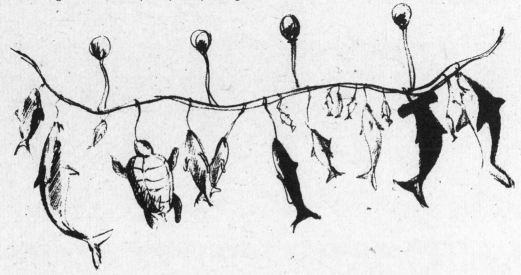

Blast fishing (in tropical regions) – dynamite explosions in the water that stun nearby fish, rupturing their bladders, which causes them to float to the surface. This highly lucrative practice destroys coral reefs, oyster beds, and productive marine habitats.

Industrial fishing destroys our oceans, injures and kills tons of bycatch and coral reefs, creating big holes in the ocean. This is causing ocean acidification. If the ocean is responsible for creating 50 per cent of the oxygen we breathe and also absorbs many greenhouse gases, it's clear that industrial fishing is damaging our health and the planet.

This sucks, buts it's a reality I'm facing with you. Can we go back to artisanal fishing? And how could we ever restore what has already been destroyed? According to the author Dr Richard Oppenlander there is no form of sustainable fishing.

FISHING SUSTAINABILITY FACTS

* *Whales die slowly trying to untangle themselves from the nets they get caught in.*
* *Sharks kill twelve people per year. We kill approximately 11,000 sharks per hour!*
* *Fish farming pollutes the oceans and fresh waters, damaging coral reefs and other oceanic populations.*
* *All ocean life, mammals such as whales, dolphins and turtles, including many endangered species, get caught and killed during routine fishing and are treated as waste.*
* *According to WWF, the global fishing industry is 2–3 times larger than the oceans can sustainably support.*
* *53 per cent of the world's fisheries are fully exploited, 32 per cent are overexploited, depleted, or recovering from depletion.*
* *Many fish and seafood are overfished. Some take a long time to mature and are often caught before they have had a chance to reproduce.*
* *Experts estimate we have removed as much as 90 per cent of the large predatory fish, including swordfish, cod, bluefin tuna and sharks from our oceans.*
* *Lost or damaged fishing gear is often left in the ocean and continues to do damage, catching and harming animals. This is known as "ghost fishing" and it is extremely destructive and wasteful.*

14 FISH WE SHOULD AVOID

Wild salmon: wild Atlantic salmon is an endangered species (and considered illegal to fish at specific periods of the year), so be careful when buying.

Farmed salmon: is grey and has pink artificial colouring and fish odour added to it. It is dangerously rich in chemicals, antibiotics, mercury, artificial colouring and now pesticides.

Farmed eel: high in PCBs and mercury.

King mackerel: high in mercury.

Orange roughy: high in mercury and overfished.

Chilean sea bass: high in mercury and overfished.

Shark: high in mercury.

Shrimp: contains high levels of antibiotics and chemical residue.

Swordfish: one of the highest in mercury, fished using long line, harming other endangered species.

Tuna (especially bluefin tuna): high in mercury and overfished, cheaper varieties can contain carbon monoxide (from colouring).

Atlantic cod: overfished.

Atlantic flatfish (sole, halibut, flounder): high in heavy metals and overfished.

Caviar: sturgeon and beluga are almost extinct.

Imported catfish: contains dangerous illegal antibiotics.

|103|

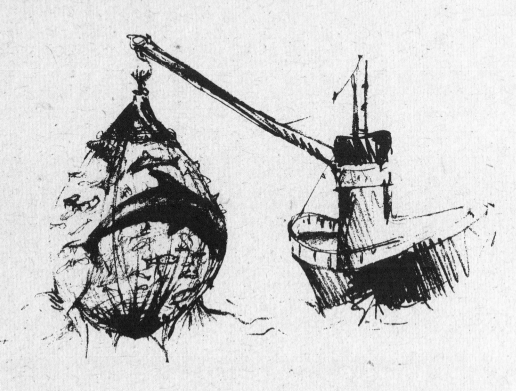

SCIENCE PROVES THAT A PLANT-BASED DIET IS A HEALTHIER CHOICE

The China Study, by T. Colin Campbell, PhD and Thomas M. Campbell, MD, proved that cultures that eat a primarily plant-based diet have lower to no instances of diseases like heart disease, diabetes, or cancer, and that switching to a plant-based diet can successfully reverse diseases already recognized in the body. The China Study is known as the most comprehensive nutritional study ever conducted on the relationship between diet and disease. This study was revolutionary for nutrition science as it was one of the first times a whole community was studied and controlled in depth. The documentary *Forks over Knives* takes you through the study itself; it's great, watch it!

As a preventative measure, finding a balance to reduce or even eliminate animal protein and its derivatives has many benefits for our bodies and the survival of our species on this planet.

JUNK-FOOD VEGETARIANS

Just because it's vegetarian or vegan doesn't mean it's healthy!

Being vegetarian or vegan is not synonymous with health. It is very easy and possible to be a junk-food vegetarian. French fries, cookies, pasta, cheese, ketchup, soft drinks and beer are all vegetarian!

REDUCE OR ELIMINATE? THAT IS THE QUESTION

Reducing or eliminating our animal intake is no doubt beneficial for our health. Numerous athletes and knowledgeable scientists, specialized doctors like oncologists and cardiologists, choose a plant-based diet for obvious reasons apart from vitality and quality of life. Some include Bill Goldberg, vegetarian athlete and world champion pro wrestler, Veronesi, an Italian oncologist who lived to be 103 years of age, Dr Caldwell Esselstyn, an American doctor, author and former Olympic rowing champion, Dr Ellsworth Wareham, a 100-year old, recently retired heart surgeon who has been a vegan for half of his life and, finally, the great Mr Einstein and Dr Darwin.

"The protein in animal products is filled with unwanted toxins, chemicals and all sorts of stuff that's harmful to you. When I was competing and stuffing down all of that, I had lots of digestive problems. I was constipated and bloated, just miserable all the time. I don't concern myself with protein anymore, because there is enough in what I eat. I am not only healthy, but I feel better about myself and how I relate to other creatures in the world."

Jim Morris, vegan body-builder

With increasing scientific evidence, medical research and personal experience, it's literally impossible to deny the fact that eating less meat is a good choice. Whether you cut it out completely or make it an occasional food for pleasure, it will always be a positive change to reduce your meat and animal consumption for your own body, your mind, and this planet.

"When it comes to getting protein in your diet, meat isn't the only option. Mounting evidence shows that reducing meat and increasing plant-based protein is a healthier way to go. A diet with any type of meat raises the risk of heart disease and cancer, when compared with a vegetarian diet."

Dr Deepak Bhatt, Harvard Medical School professor and editor-in-chief of the Harvard Heart Letter

Consider yourself challenged

* Meat is not essential for vitality or health.

* The consumption of animal products has been linked to a long list of diseases, including the top killers in today's world and the top five cancers. Science has proved the health benefits of a vegetarian or plant-based diet.

* All processes involved in feeding, raising, slaughtering and transporting animal foods including dairy, eggs and meat cause more than 40 per cent of greenhouses gasses. Overfishing has depleted the oceans that absorb 50 per cent of the very greenhouse gasses we're producing. So, we are increasing the gasses and destroying the ocean that helps to remove these gasses.

So, if it's not essential for vitality or health, it's actually less healthy than we thought, and now we know it's devastating for the environment, let's be honest with ourselves: do we need to eat as much meat and animal products as we do? I hereby present a challenge:

1. Reduce the amount of animal products you eat by more than 60 per cent.

2. Introduce new alternatives to dairy, eggs, fish and meat. For example: **Breakfast:** a juice, almond smoothie, gluten-free granola or oats with almond milk or coconut yoghurt, or a miso soup. **Lunch/dinner:** garden curry/risotto or a veggie burger with quinoa/brown rice and salad, or a massive salad with roasted veggies, sweet potatoes, nuts and seeds with tahini dressing, yum! **Snacks:** hummus or avocado veggie wrap or sweet potato wedges with pesto dip.

3. Reduce your meat feasts to three meals a week. Make it a celebration.

   * Be wise and choose quality grass-fed, pasture-raised, organic if possible, local, and question if the animal was treated humanely.

   * Use meat as a condiment, to simply give flavour to vegetable-rich stews and beans (feijoada/dahl).

   * Have a smaller portion, the size of a card deck.

> * Be adventurous with colourful veggies and yummy beans!
>
> 4. Use the Real Food Shopping List to fill your kitchen with deliciousness and check out the meal plans (see pages 268–71) to get a good idea of what a week of meals could look like.
>
> If we fill our plates with a combination of beans, grains, vegetables, nuts, seeds and sprouts, and eat until we're satisfied, we will be getting enough protein.
>
> Are you cool enough to take this on for the benefit of your future and the future of your kids, your animals and the planet?
>
> **Secret tip:** if you add red wine and thyme to a risotto dish, it tastes like it has meat in it! Use seasoning on veggies that you would use on meat to trick your mind, because your mind is definitely the only thing getting in your way!

MorLife Wellness is about becoming more conscious. If you have never thought about the source of your nutrients and protein, animal or plant, start thinking about it. Look at your food and ask where it comes from. If you choose animal protein, make sure it's from an animal that was properly treated rather than industrially farmed and slaughtered. If it feels right to reduce the amount of animal foods you eat, be brave, creative, and remember it's not a religion so you can always vary and change your options. I do not think that meat is categorically bad. But what we have done to it, the fact that most of our meat is heavily processed, means that it IS bad for us. My advice is see meat as an occasional food; eat it when you really want to enjoy it, perhaps on a special night out or at a special event. Be respectful of the animal you are eating. Did you know that when bushmen catch their hunt they say a prayer and thank the animal for sacrificing its life to feed them? Buy good-quality meat, or find a farmer nearby that can sell you fresh meat that you can freeze and consume over a month. Find ways to bet on quality and reduce the quantity for the good of your own precious body and of the planet!

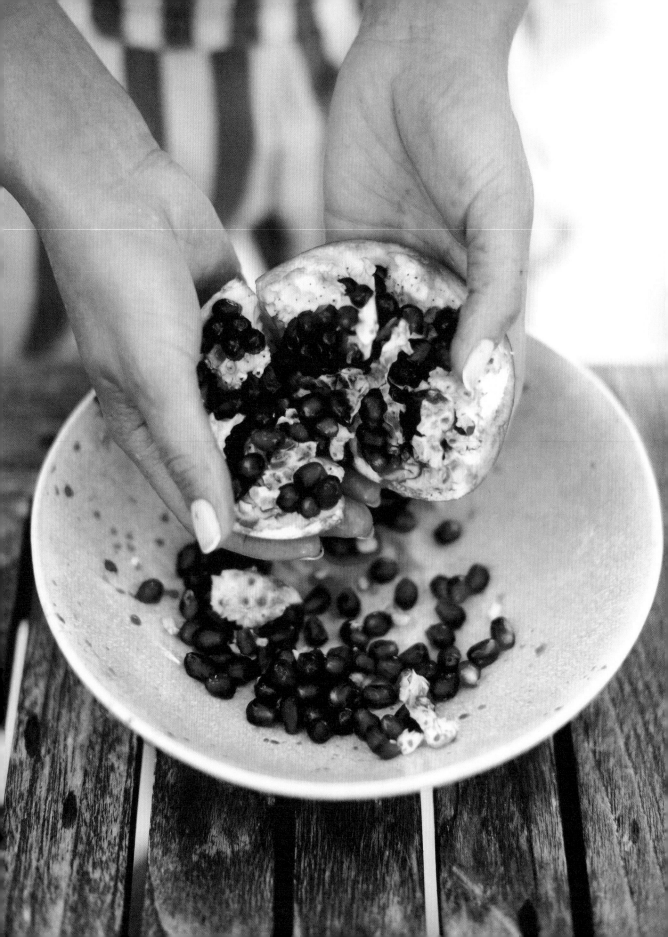

*Our body
is alkaline
by design,
and acid
by function.*

Chapter 6

ALKALIZE
FIRST

BALANCE YOUR BODY

THE PH BALANCE OF THE HUMAN BLOODSTREAM IS ONE OF THE MOST IMPORTANT BIO-CHEMICAL BALANCES FOR HEALTH. WE CONTROL OUR BODY'S PH WITH OUR DAILY CHOICES, FROM FOOD AND LIFESTYLE, TO ACTIONS AND THOUGHTS.

Alkaline is the opposite of acid. pH balance determines whether something is an acid (pH lower than 7) or an alkaline (pH higher than 7). All life on earth depends on the correct pH levels – both in and around living organisms.

Everything from healthy cells to cancer cells to soil quality and ocean life is affected by pH. The health of our bodies, skin, hair, organs and immune response is linked to maintaining the perfect pH balance.

Think of the pH balance as a basic need for anything to function. Imagine an office with lots of people working at their desks. We can say that a comfortable temperature is a basic need. If it were below zero degrees, people would probably find it hard to do their normal work. And if it were far below freezing, they would likely be so destabilized by the external freezing temperature that they would become dysfunctional.

This is similar to the pH balance within us. If our body, or part of our body, becomes a different pH to what it should be, it doesn't function correctly. The acidification of our oceans is similarly destabilizing the ocean's capacity to properly function and offer the best environment for marine life – and this puts our oceans and lives at great risk. When we mess with pH balance, we are messing with the ability for survival.

pH imbalance can explain many health disorders, and that's why it's an important step toward vitality and why it's part of this book!

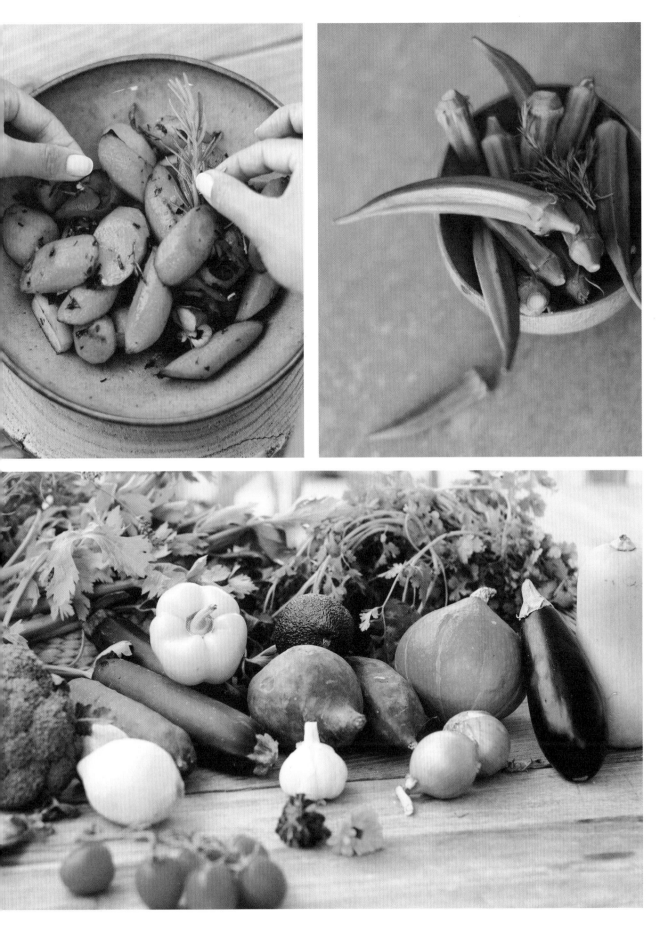

ALKALINE BODY

Our body functions at its best in a mildly alkaline state. This means that the foods we eat and the water and liquids we drink should encourage alkalinity. Bacteria, viruses, fungi and any other inflammation or infection – even cancer cells – proliferate in an acidic environment.

When you make the same environment alkaline, unwanted organisms and cells die. Noble prize-winner Dr Otto H Warburg said, "No disease, including cancer, can exist in an alkaline environment."

THE PH SCALE

ACID   NEUTRAL   ALKALINE

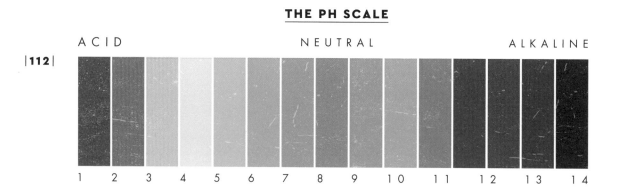

1   2   3   4   5   6   7   8   9   10   11   12   13   14

ACID BODY

When our body becomes more acidic, it is the perfect environment for bacterial growth, cancer cell multiplication, and all forms of infection and inflammation to get out of hand. Even if you are already ill or infected, by drastically creating an alkaline environment, you can feel better quite quickly because you are literally killing the *baddies*.

If it's that simple, why isn't everyone living an alkaline lifestyle?

HOW WE BECOME ACIDIC

Our body is a bag of chemical reactions. Our thoughts, actions, lifestyle, the foods we eat and whatever we absorb or inhale becomes chemistry. When we eat a steak, the final product in our bodies causes acidity, making this food an acid-forming food. Negative self-talk and thoughts produce acid chemicals in the brain, which spread acidity throughout the body. Not only can we become acidic through stress and eating certain foods, the chemicals in our environment, our cosmetics, our detergents and other household products can also cause acidic imbalances in our bodies.

When this happens, our bodies work hard to redress the balance and recruit alkaline minerals like calcium, magnesium, and potassium from our bones, teeth and organs to balance and neutralize the acidity in the body! *What?* In other words when we get too acidic, from the acid-forming food we eat or negative emotions and stress, our body literally steals minerals from our bones to neutralize the acidity in our blood. This reduces the quality of our bones. **Our blood's pH is slightly alkaline at approximately 7.365. The harder it has to work to maintain this level the more stress it causes on the body.**

SIGNS OF AN ACIDIC BODY

Fatigue is the first sign of acidity in the body!

* *Skin eruptions*
* *Headaches*
* *Allergies*
* *Colds and flu*
* *Sinus problems*
* *Inflammatory conditions*

An acidic pH imbalance in the body has been linked with several conditions. These include:
* *Excessive weight gain/weight loss*
* *Mood disorders*
* *Neurological imbalances*
* *Allergies and food intolerances*
* *Inflammation*
* *Skin problems*
* *Constipation*
* *Bowel issues*
* *Stress (physical and mental)*
* *Arthritis*
* *Chronic disease*
* *Diabetes*
* *Cholesterol*
* *Cancerous cells*
* *Osteoporosis*
* *Hindered kidney function*

If you have any of the above, this chapter is a perfect starting point.

Acidity reveals itself in six stages in our bodies:

* Loss of energy, fatigue
* Sensitivity and irritation (IBS)
* Mucus and congestion
* Inflammation
* Hardening of soft tissue
* Degeneration – cancer, heart disease, stroke, MS, diabetes, etc.

"Physiological disease is almost always the result of too much acid stressing the body's pH balance."

Dr Young, pH expert

CAN WE BE TOO ALKALINE?

It would be hard to become too alkaline in our wonderful industrial world. The high level of acid-forming pollutants, stress and chemicals we are exposed to daily, not to mention our food choices, means it's likely most of us are acidic and that's why we're tired and constipated.

THOUGHTS, EMOTIONS AND PH

Stress, sadness, anger, revenge, irritation, depression and negative thoughts create acidity through brain chemistry and can be worse than eating acidic-forming foods. Making an effort to create a positive mindset and focusing on positivity in your life will benefit your body and, in turn, your mind. See Chapter 13 (pages 232–53).

Interesting FACT!

Healthy cells in the body thrive in mild, moderate, and high pH fluids. They lose function in even a mild acidic state. Cancerous (and harmful) cells, on the other hand, thrive in an acidic pH of 5.5. They become dormant at an alkaline pH of 7.365 or higher, and die at a pH of 8.5, while healthy cells live!

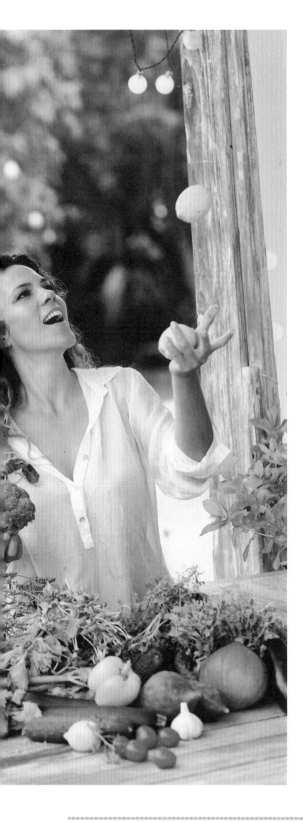

AN ALKALINE DIET

An alkaline diet can help increase weight loss, stop allergies, hyperactivity and ADD/ADHD.

When the body is too acidic, it creates fat cells to store excess acids in an effort to protect our vital organs from becoming overly acidic – our fat can actually save our lives! However, this is why our body doesn't want to let go of it. By alkalizing the body, the fat is no longer needed and, as a result, fat will melt away, along with its acidic contents. A healthy body will naturally maintain its ideal weight.

I suffered from chronic rhinitis and started noticing it was linked to when I ate acid-forming foods, especially sugary foods in the evening. I have since significantly controlled my allergies by being more alkaline with both my dietary and lifestyle choices, and being allergy-free has definitely been worth it!

Eat, drink, move and think in ways that recreate the body's alkaline nature.

HOW TO ALKALIZE

ALKALIZE SMART

I have my kitchen set up so that alkaline foods are the easiest to find. I do my shopping according to the alkaline charts (see right). Hang 'em on your fridge or wherever you can easily see them. I leave the acidic foods for when I'm out with friends. For example, I don't shop for bread. It's an occasional food, which I can have when I really feel like a baguette or a croissant. I don't shop for desserts. I leave those for the outings in town with friends.

ALKALINE FIRST

My trick is to crowd out. When I'm hungry, I choose "alkaline foods first" so that I devour foods that are better for my body. Once I've relaxed from hunger, I can enjoy the rest, but since I'm already slightly filled, I won't eat as much. This is a smart way to start any meal. When I was growing up, we always had a big salad with a delicious dressing on the table before the hot meal was served. I remember being so hungry that I would eat anything. Sometimes I ate so much salad I wasn't even hungry for the meal.

80/20

"Alkaline first" is really simple and easy to apply. 80 per cent of what you eat can be alkalizing: fresh, energizing vegetables, salads, seeds and nuts, and only 20 per cent acid-forming foods such as pizza, dairy, alcohol, fizzy drinks, meats, and so on. Minimize your consumption of these acid-forming foods; leave them for occasional events. Aim for an 80/20 ratio of alkaline/acid.

ACID/ALKALINE FOOD CHARTS

The charts on the following pages are perfect for an overall understanding of how acid or alkaline foods play out in the body. Lemons and apple cider vinegar are acid-tasting but super alkalizing in the body! Sugar, although it tastes sweet, is very acid-forming – in fact, anything sweet, including sweet fruits, are more acid-forming. Stick to less sweet fruits like avocados, green apples, pears and pomegranates. You'll find that these charts are very handy to refer back to, so why not cut them out and stick them on your fridge?

THE MORLIFE ACID/ALKALINE FOOD CHART

< EAT MORE   EAT LESS >

HIGHLY ALKALINE	MODERATELY ALKALINE	MILDLY ALKALINE	NEUTRAL/MILDLY ACIDIC	MODERATELY ACIDIC	HIGHLY ACIDIC
Broccoli	Avocado	Artichokes	Black Beans	Fresh, Natural Juice	Alcohol
Cucumber	Beetroot	Asparagus	Brazil nuts	Ketchup	Coffee & Black tea
Grasses	Capsicum/Pepper	Brussels Sprouts	Cantaloupe	Mayonnaise	Fruit Juice (sweetened)
Himalayan Salt	Cabbage	Buckwheat	Chickpeas	Butter	Cocoa
Kale	Celery	Cauliflower	Currants	Apple	Honey
Parsley	Collard/Spring Greens	Carrot	Kidney Beans	Apricot	Jam
Spinach	Endive	Coconut	Seitan	Banana	Jelly
All Sprouted Beans	Garlic	Courgette (Zucchini)	Fresh Dates	Blackberry	Mustard
Sprouts (alfalfa etc)	Ginger	Goat and Almond Milk	Nectarine	Blueberry	Miso
Sea Vegetables (kelp)	Green Beans	Grapefruit	Plum	Cranberry	Rice Syrup
	Lettuce	Herbs and Spices	Sweet Cherry	Grapes	Soy Sauce
	Mustard Greens	Leeks	Watermelon	Mango	Vinegar
	Okra	Lentils	Amaranth	Mangosteen	Yeast
	Onion	New Potatoes	Millet	Orange	Dried Fruit
	Radish	Olives	Oats/Oatmeal	Peach	Beef
	Red Onion	Peas	Spelt	Papaya	Chicken
	Rocket/Arugula	Pomegranate	Soybeans	Pineapple	Eggs
	Tomato	Pumpkin	Rice/Soy/Hemp	Strawberry	Farmed Fish
	Lemon	Rhubarb	Freshwater/Wild Fish	Brown Rice	Pork
	Lime	Swede (Rutabaga)	Rice and Soy Milk	Oat	Shellfish
	Butter (Lima) Beans	Sweet Potato	Pecan Nuts	Rye Bread	Cheese
	Soy Beans	Squash	Hazelnuts	Wheat	Dairy
	White Haricot Beans	Watercress	Sunflower Oil	Wholemeal Bread	Artificial Sweeteners
	Chia/Salba		Grapeseed Oil	Wild Rice	Syrup
	Quinoa			Wholemeal Pasta	Mushrooms
				Ocean Fish	

THE DETAILED LIST OF ALKALINE FOODS

VEGETABLES

Asparagus	Chives	Cucumber
Broccoli	Endive	Watercress
Chilli	Chard	Lettuce
Capsicum/	Cabbage	Peas
Pepper	Sweet Potato	Broad Beans
Courgette/	Coriander	New Potato
Zucchini	Basil	Pumpkin
Dandelion	Brussels Sprouts	Radish
Snowpeas	Cauliflower	Squashes
Green Beans	Carrot	(summer,
String Beans	Beetroot	butternut etc)
Runner Beans	Eggplant/	Turnip
Spinach	Aubergine	
Kale	Garlic	
Wakame	Onion	
Kelp	Parsley	
Collards	Celery	

FRUITS

Avocado
Tomato
Lemon
Lime
Grapefruit
Fresh Coconut
Pomegranate
Melon
Kiwi

GRAINS &BEANS

Amaranth
Buckwheat
Brown Rice
Chia/Salba
Kamut
Millet
Quinoa
Spelt
Lentils
Lima Beans
Mung Beans
Navy Beans
Pinto Beans
Red Beans
Soy Beans
White Beans

SPROUTS

All Sprouted Beans
(Lentils, Mung, Adzuki)
Alfalfa Sprouts
Amaranth Sprouts
Broccoli Sprouts
Fenugreek Sprouts

NUTS &SEEDS

Almonds
Coconut
Flax Seeds
Pumpkin Seeds
Sesame Seeds
Sunflower Seeds

BREADS

Sprouted Bread
Sprouted Wraps
Gluten/Yeast Free
Breads & Wraps

GRASSES

Wheatgrass
Barley Grass
Kamut Grass
Oat Grass

OILS

Avocado Oil
Coconut Oil
Flax Oil
Olive Oil

OTHER

Alkaline Water
Goat & Almond Milk
Herbal Tea
Buckwheat Pasta

THE DETAILED LIST OF ACID FOODS

MEAT
Bacon
Beef
Clams
Corned Beef
Eggs
Lamb
Lobster
Mussels
Organ Meats
Venison
Fish
Oyster
Pork
Rabbit
Sausage
Scallops
Shellfish
Shrimp
Tuna
Turkey
Veal

FRUITS
Apple
Apricot
Currants
Dates
Grapes
Mango
Peach
Pear
Prunes
Raisins
Raspberries
Strawberries
Tropical Fruits
Berries
Cantaloupe
Cranberries
Currants
Honeydew
Melon
Orange
Pineapple
Plum

DRINKS
Alcohol
Black Tea
Coffee
Carbonated Water
Pasteurized Juice
Cocoa
Energy Drinks
Sports Drinks
Colas
Tap Water
Milk
Green Tea
Decaffeinated Drinks
Flavoured Water

DAIRY & EGGS
Butter
Cheese
Milk
Whey
Yogurt
Cottage Cheese
Ice Cream
Sour Cream
Soy Cheese
Eggs

SWEETENERS
Artificial Sweeteners
Carob
Corn Syrup
Fructose
Processed Sugar
Saccharine
Sucrose
Sucralose
Honey
Maple Syrup

NUTS & SEEDS
Cashews
Peanuts
Pecans
Pistachios
Walnuts
Brazil Nuts
Chestnuts
Hazelnuts
Macadamia Nuts

SAUCES
Mayonnaise
Ketchup
Mustard
Soy Sauce
Pickles
Vinegar
Tabasco
Tamari
Wasabi

OILS
Cooked Oil
Solid Oil (Margarine)
Oil Exposed to heat, light or air

OTHER
Mushrooms
Miso
White Breads
Pastas
Rice & Noodles
Chocolate
Chips
Pizza
Biscuits
Cigarettes
Drugs
Candy!

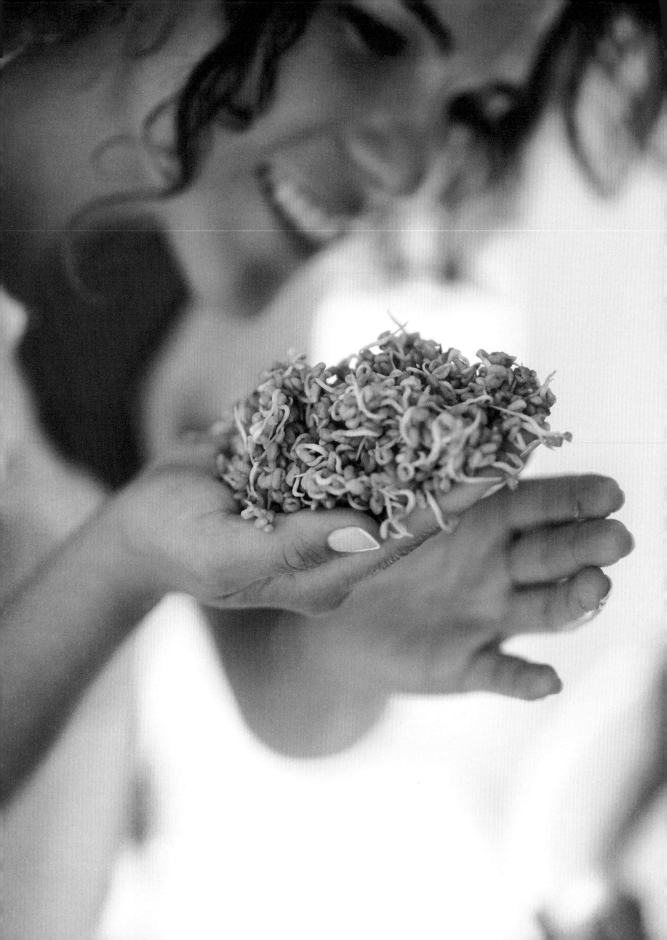

> *Money may make the world go round, but without enzymes, life doesn't exist. So, between us, get rich on enzymes.*

Chapter 7

GET RICH ON ENZYMES

EAT YOURSELF YOUNG

AS WE AGE, WE USE UP OUR ENZYME SUPPLY; AGEING IS ACTUALLY A RESULT OF DECREASING ENZYME CONCENTRATIONS IN THE BODY. THE MORE WE DEPLETE OUR ENZYMES, THE MORE WE DAMAGE AND DESTABILIZE OUR BODY, WEAKEN OUR IMMUNE SYSTEM AND AGE QUICKER. ABOVE ALL, WE REDUCE OUR QUALITY OF LIFE, WHICH IS PRICELESS. NOW DO YOU GET WHY GETTING RICH ON ENZYMES IS THE SECRET TO LONGEVITY?

Understanding how enzymes work helped me realize just how important it is to eat more of nature's food in its natural state.

Processing foods in any way, even cooking them, significantly kills the enzymes and makes a food less nutritious.

OUR ENZYME BANK ACCOUNT

Our enzyme supply works in a similar way to a savings account. Our daily body functions make withdrawals from our enzyme account. When we eat real food in its natural form, uncooked and naturally rich in enzymes, we make deposits into our enzyme account. Our enzyme levels require constant topping up through our food.

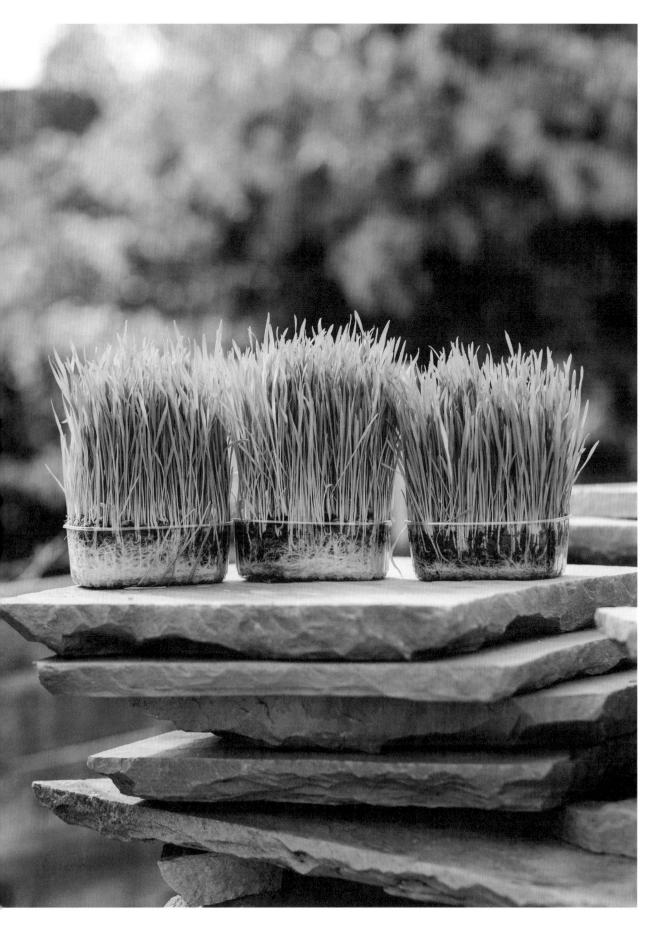

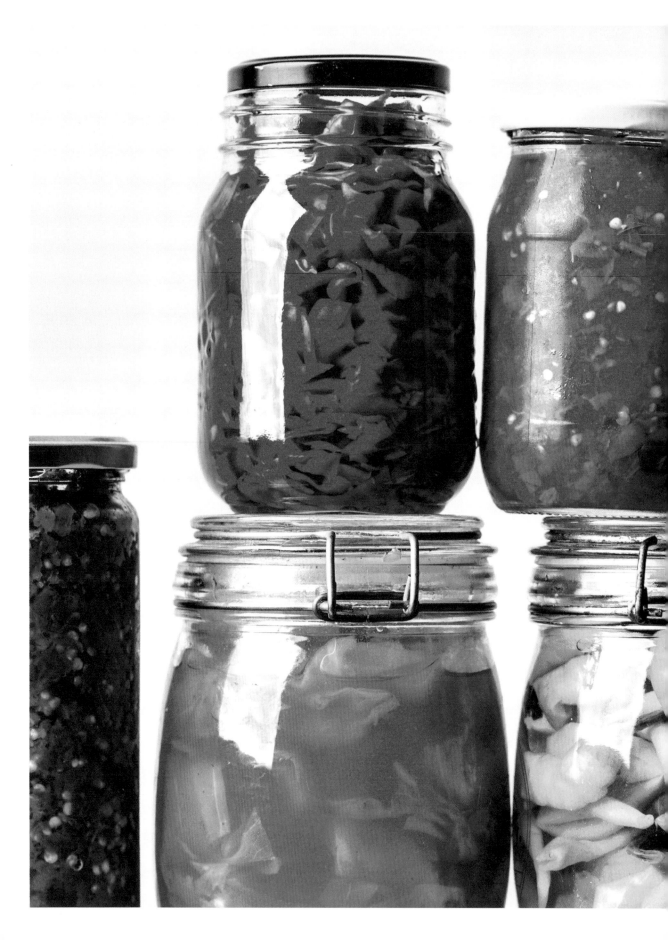

WHAT ARE ENZYMES?

Enzymes are proteins. They activate and carry out all biological and biochemical processes in the body. Every single reaction in our body depends on enzymes! Without them, we cannot exist. Perhaps you have heard about enzymes having an important role in digestion – these babies are not only crucial for digestion, but fundamental to our complete existence! If low enzyme count causes indigestion, imagine what they cause in our circulatory and immune systems.

When we eat food with little or no enzymes, our body uses our enzyme stocks for digestion, which slows down enzyme supply to the brain, circulatory system, immune system, and more.

WHAT WE NEED TO KNOW: 4 KEY CONCEPTS

The topic of enzymes is super intricate. I have simplified it for us.

1. Enzymes are crucial for life and are responsible for:

* *Digestion*
* *Transmitting nerve impulses*
* *Muscle movement*
* *Detoxification*
* *DNA/RNA functioning*
* *Repair and healing of the body*
* *Every function from blinking and thinking to chewing and pooing!*

2. The capacity of an organism to make enzymes is exhaustible. This means we can slowly run out of them, which is what happens when we don't replenish our enzyme stock. *Enzymes die at high temperatures, at 42°C. That's why we feel sluggish with a fever, when our enzymes become less efficient.*

3. Enzymes die when food is cooked, processed, pasteurized or radiated. So, a highly nutritious food like milk loses its nutritional value when pasteurized. Its nutrition and abundant enzymes die.

4. An alkaline body is the best environment for these life sparks to work their magic! In an acidic body, you can feel lethargic and sick and have brain fog because your enzymes are less efficient. So alkalize, baby!

ENZYME-RICH FOOD SOURCES (NATURE'S REAL SUPERFOODS)

Enzyme-rich foods are loaded with enzymes and nutrients, which help with their own digestion and top up your enzyme account. These include:

* Sprouts (germinated seeds, nuts, beans and grains)
* Fermented, unpasteurized foods – sauerkraut, kimchi, kefir, etc.
* Fresh, uncooked vegetables, fruits, sea- and fresh-water algae (eaten as close to harvesting as possible, as enzymes slowly die once the plant is removed or cut from its natural habitat).

"The only natural source of enzymes is raw plant-based food."

Brian Clement, PhD, author of Food IS Medicine

SPROUTS: THE MOST ENZYME-RICH FOOD

What are sprouts? The miracle of life! A sprout is a germinated seed, grain, bean, legume or nut. When a seed germinates, an incredible flow of energy is released. Natural chemical charges occur, enzymes are produced, and all nutrients are converted into the most easily digestible molecules for the seed to grow into a large plant or tree. When we eat sprouts, our body is flooded with these easily digestible nutrients. Sprouts are biogenic and capable of creating life! When eaten, they transfer their life energy to your body. It's pretty amazing, I think!

Sprouts are living foods. They are literally growing as you bite into them, or as they chill in your sandwich 'til lunch!

Living food has HOPE:

H - Hormones
O - Oxygen
P - Phytonutrients
E - Enzymes

These hormones help keep the inner communications of the body strong and prevent disruption!

Sprouts are nature's multivitamins. They offer the most concentrated, easily absorbed and natural forms of vitamins, minerals, enzymes and amino-acids (proteins) known to man.

Sprouts grown from nuts, seeds, grains and beans contain 10–30 times more concentrated nutrients than many vegetables. Some are 35 per cent protein (a higher percentage than many animal foods).

How to eat your sprouts:

It's easy and fun to grow sprouts, but getting them into your meals is the challenge!

1. Add them into sandwiches.

2. Mix them into your salad, sushi rolls, or stuff them into a wrap.

3. Fold them into omelettes, quesadillas or burritos.

4. Add them to your stir-fry, soup or curry just before serving (don't cook them so you can absorb their life force and nutrients).

5. You can also sprout beans and legumes before cooking them to make bean casseroles, soups and hummus. This increases their nutrient bioavailability, protein level and digestibility (they're no longer gas-producing, for example!)

Be creative!

BENEFITS OF SPROUTING

* *Nutritional value increases by more than 10 times!*
* *Increases bio-availability of proteins, vitamins, minerals and antioxidants, so they are absorbed more easily into the body*
* *Increases the availability of calcium, iron and zinc*
* *Increases fibre content*
* *Sprouting grains breaks down gluten for easier digestibility*
* *Helps reduce other allergens found in grains*
* *Increases enzymes and antioxidants*
* *Inexpensive and easy to grow*
* *Vitamin and nutrient-dense food source all year round, especially in winter!*
* *Practical process (homegrown fresh produce)*
* *Adds texture to meals and salads!*

Sprouts are a unique superfood with potent medicinal qualities. They are essentially a high-quality, low-cost multivitamin, extremely rich in:

* *Vitamin C*
* *Vitamin B1, B2, B3, B5, B6*
* *Carotene*
* *Vitamins A, D, E and K*
* *Calcium*
* *Carbohydrates*
* *Chlorophyll*
* *Iron*
* *Magnesium*
* *Niacin*
* *Phosphorus*
* *Potassium*
* *All essential amino acids*
* *Trace elements, such as iodine, zinc, selenium, chromium, cobalt and silicon*

LOW COST – HIGH QUALITY

Sprouting is a perfect option for low-cost high-nutrient meals. In fact, researchers say that sprouts could be used to solve human deficiency problems worldwide and in developing countries.

You can buy sprouts or grow your own in your kitchen! A combination of sprouts will give you the recommended daily allowance of protein, vitamins and minerals – all inexpensive and homegrown, organic and natural, even in the winter! Seeds and beans are cheap, and yield crazy amounts of sprouts. One handful of beans yields four handfuls of sprouts!

Sprouting is easy and fun; the challenge is creating a sprouting routine. And, of course, eating them is the important part! Be courageous and check out the "How to Sprout" section (page 130). If you have kids, get them involved. They love watching things grow.

STAY HEALTHY WITH SPROUTS!

SPROUT NAME	HEALTH BENEFIT
Fenugreek seeds – the heartiest of all sprouts	Creates a medicinal gel that helps combat diabetes, common digestive disorders and body odour.
Mung beans (Chinese bean sprouts) – the most easily digestible food	Their potent zinc content, other minerals, and digestible proteins can help prevent prostate problems, glandular dysfunction and breast cancer, as well as premature balding and greying.
Lentils	Rich in all vitamins especially vitamin C – a powerful antioxidant that also builds the protein collagen necessary for the production of blood vessels, cartilage, ligaments, skin and tendons as well as the repair and maintenance of teeth and bones.
Almonds, hazelnuts, macadamia, pine nuts, pistachios	Rich in protein and essential fatty acids, strengthens cells, builds muscle structure, and sustains the heart.
Sunflower and pea greens: Sunflower and pea sprouts may be grown on soil or hydroponically in nutritionally enriched pure water for seven days.	Both these baby greens are considered the most balanced of all the sources of essential amino acids. They are a perfect source of complete protein and essential fatty acids; they activate every cell in the immune system, and build skeletal, muscular and the neurological systems; they are also powerful sources of antioxidants, minerals, vitamins and enzymes that protect against free radical damage.

HOW TO SPROUT

Buy seeds in bulk and store them for long periods of time without spoilage. Store them in airtight containers, in a dark and cool place away from heat and sunlight. If you live in a hot country it's best to freeze them. This keeps them safe! I find fenugreek and mung beans to be the most available and easiest to sprout. If they are not available in health-food stores, you can always find them in Indian food stores.

Growing your own sprouts is the new cool! Inexpensive and super easy to grow, sprouts are one of the most economically sustainable foods you can grow on your kitchen countertop at any time of the year. They are the true foods of the future.

LET'S SPROUT!

Tools and Resources
* Colander/sieve/jar
* Plate
* Water
* Sprouting subject

Use raw, unroasted, un-blanched grains, beans, nuts, seeds or legumes. Ensure they are not irradiated.

1. Soak seeds for 24–48 hours in a bowl, immersed and covered with several centimetres of filtered water. Each day, drain, rinse and change the water for fresh water. (Notice how much they have enlarged!)

2. After 24–48 hours place the seeds in a sieve, colander, sprouting bag or jar without any water. (Should be humid, not dry.)

3. Rinse sprouts 3x daily with fresh water to keep them humid and clean of mould (before work or school, after work and before bed, for example).

4. Repeat the process until the sprouts have a 0.5cm tail. (Ensure the sprouts don't dry up. Keep them humid.)

5. With a tail of 0.5cm, sprouts are ready to eat!
Eat me! Rinse ready-to-eat sprouts with fresh water and serve in salads, wraps, smoothies, juices, on breads/crackers, or just eat as a snack.
Storing tips: Let dry and then refrigerate for up to one week. Always rinse sprouts before eating, as they are growing just like us and they eliminate waste and toxins.

I like to be adventurous with sprouting. Experiment and find out which are your favourites. If you buy organic seeds you can grow organic food for pennies.

I love sprouting. It's fun to see them grow a little more each day.

Watching how simple nature is, really is so incredible. These seeds are dormant and then suddenly, just because we add water and oxygen, they become lifeforces and grow into a mother plant! Now, don't be like me and forget them in the fridge... only to remember a week later when they are already dried up. Stick the "How to eat your sprouts" list onto your fridge so you actually eat them!

Nuts

All raw nuts can be sprouted. Reduce or avoid peanut consumption as they are high in toxins.

Sprouting nuts such as almonds and hazelnuts can makes their nutrients more bio-available. Here's how:

Soak them overnight, then place them on an unbleached paper towel and spray them with pure water at least two times daily. They will be ready to eat around the third day. Sprouted nuts are alive and therefore need to be eaten within a few days.

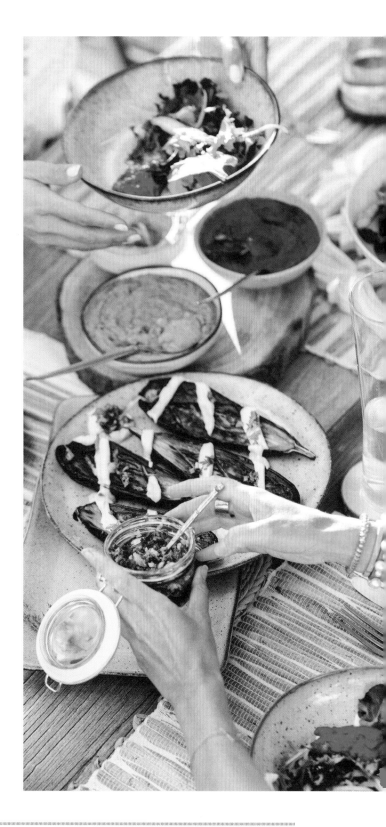

IS YOUR FOOD ENZYME-RICH?

How alive and enzyme-rich is the food you're eating? Since the industrialization of food, most of our food comes packaged, tinned, frozen or pre-cooked. Unfortunately, this convenience has stolen nutrients from our food and bodies. The secret to topping up our enzyme account is to eat foods in their natural state, raw and uncooked.

Nature created foods with super-powers to feed you, the superhero.

SUPERFOODS FOR SUPERHEROES

Superfoods / su:pəfu:d,sju:-/
A nutrient-rich food considered to be exceptionally beneficial for health.

Many foods are casually referred to as "superfoods", such as oats and berries, to an extent that it has become a fashion. These foods are healthy, but their superfood claims are usually exaggerated for marketing reasons. Let's remember the real superfoods on this planet! A superfood has an exceptional number of vitamins, minerals, phytonutrients, enzymes and antioxidants. It's a highly nutrient-dense food with exceptional nutritional value and multiple health benefits.

Superfoods from the land: sprouts, baby greens, wheatgrass, micro sunflower greens, pea greens

Superfoods from the sea and freshwater lakes: green and green/blue algae, spirulina, chlorella, AFA (Aphanizomenon flos-aquae)
Note: what these foods have in common is their unique ability to transform sunlight energy into edible energy. Eating these organisms equals eating pure sunshine! Just like eating leafy greens.

Superfoods are a class of the most potent, concentrated and nutrient-rich foods on the planet. Tasty and satisfying, superfoods have the ability to seriously increase the vital lifeforce and energy of your body. They boost the immune system, increase serotonin production, potentialize libido, cleanse and alkalize the body, enhancing enzymatic efficiency and protecting it from pathogens. These superfoods ultimately nourish us at the deepest level possible. They are the true fuel of today's "superhero". Superfoods are packed with enzymes!

THE WHEATGRASS SHOT

Wheatgrass is a powerful raw, living superfood, containing over a hundred easily absorbable nutrients, including thirteen essential vitamins, all existing minerals known to man, numerous trace elements, seventeen amino acids (including the essential nine) and over eighty enzymes! Wheatgrass is also one of the richest sources of chlorophyll on the planet. Chlorophyll, the green pigment, is what holds most of the nutrition.

INTERESTING FACT: 60ml of wheatgrass juice has the nutritional equivalent of 2.5kg of the best raw organic vegetables.

"Wheatgrass juice is the most potent and accessible purifier known to man."

Dr Brian Clement, PhD, author of Living Foods for Optimum Health

Wheatgrass is:
* An excellent source of protein, with about 20 per cent of total calories coming from protein.
* This protein is more absorbable than animal protein.
* Extremely rich in vitamins, minerals, antioxidants, enzymes and phytonutrients.
* A powerful detoxifier (especially of the liver and blood).
* Helps neutralize toxins and environmental pollutants in the body.
* Cleanses the body of heavy metals, pollutants and other toxins stored in body tissues and organs.

Getting regularly drunk on wheatgrass shots can help you:
* Develop a healthy immune system.
* Detoxify the digestive tract and support intestinal health.
* Optimize a healthy circulatory system.
* Lose weight.
* Improve skin, hair and nails.
* Decrease bodily odours.
* Reduce tooth decay.
* Keep your bowel movements regular.
* Neutralize toxins.

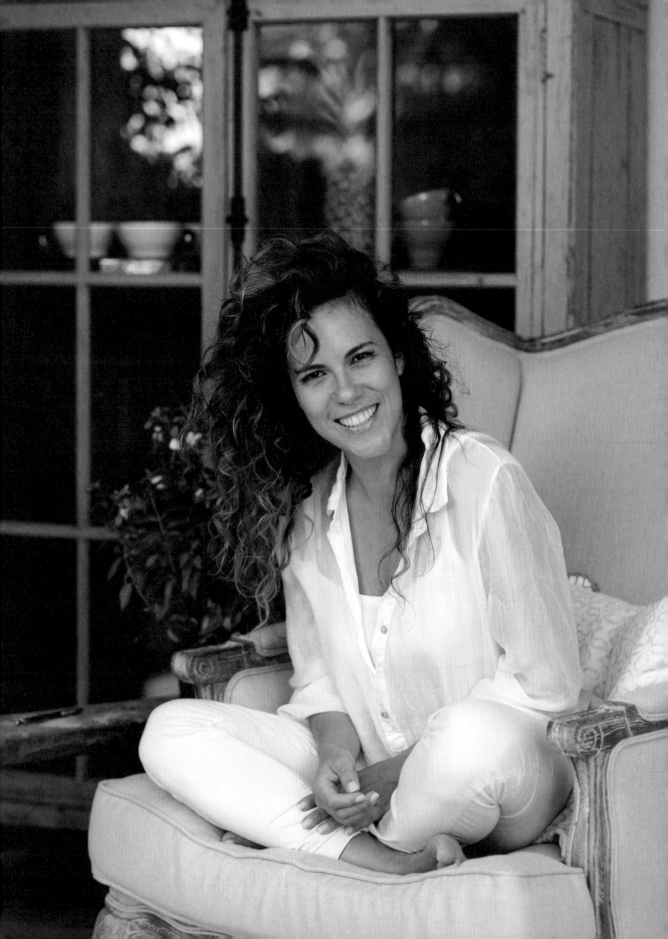

> *It's not what you do once in a while; it's what you do every day that makes the difference.*

Chapter 8

CUT THE CRAP (MOST OF THE TIME)

YOU CAN DO IT!

NOW THAT WE KNOW THERE IS SO MUCH TOXICITY IN OUR FOOD INDUSTRY, LET'S LOOK AT THE BENEFITS OF REMOVING THESE TOXIC SUBSTANCES FROM OUR LIVES. IT CAN BE AMAZING TO DISCOVER THAT YOUR LIFE CAN CHANGE BY SIMPLY REMOVING ONE TOXIC FOOD. SO MANY OF MY CLIENTS HAVE HEALED COMMON DISCOMFORTS, EVEN DISEASE, BY CUTTING THE CRAP.

This chapter is a straightforward note to anyone who wants to feel better as quickly as possible. Removing the "crap" from your daily habits will change how you feel, look and function.

Cutting the crap, the toxicity, should always be the first step toward vitality. You can eat the healthiest food but if you keep attacking your body with toxic food and toxic substances, you will never feel better.

This is a simple yet practical chapter that inspires you to have the courage to use the great tools and delicious solutions presented throughout the book. The little bit of science will help you understand why certain foods hurt our bodies, arming you with information that will strengthen your new choices and make them easier to implement into your life.

It's not what you do once in a while; it's what you do every day that makes the difference.

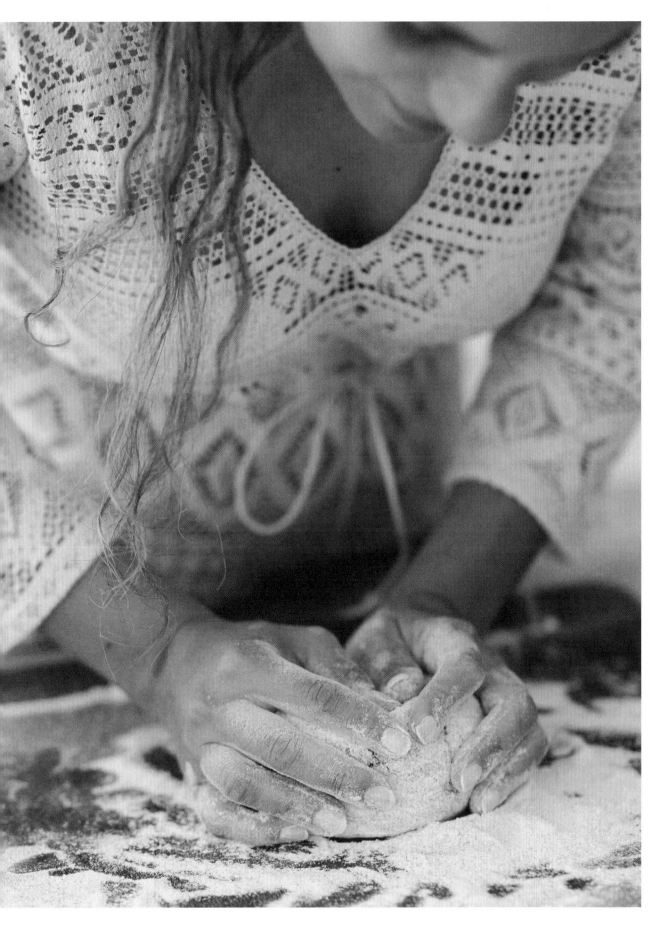

EATING NUTRIENT-RICH FOOD VS CUTTING OUT TOXIC FOOD

When it comes to health and vitality, which is more important? When someone reverses disease with a highly nutritious diet, does the body heal because of the high-quality food or because of the absence of harmful toxic food? Is it possible that by simply cutting the crap, our body can work its magic and prevent or reverse health issues?

During my studies at the Hippocrates Health Institute in Florida, where people have reversed diabetes, infertility, irritable bowel syndrome (IBS), chronic fatigue syndrome (CFS) and even cancer, we often asked ourselves this question.

The main foods that cause inflammation, irritation, mucus and congestion in the body are:
* Dairy
* Wheat and gluten
* Sugar
* Refined carbohydrates (the white fluffy foods and alcohol)
* Processed foods
* Processed meat (ham, sausages, etc.)
* Factory-farmed meat and fish

You may have a special relationship with one or more of these foods and feel that you couldn't possibly live without it. But keep reading... learning about how you could feel better than you do can be empowering. Be courageous and find out how your body might be reacting to our modern foods. Many of my clients are astonished to discover how amazing they feel by cutting just one inflammatory food from their daily life.

Several of my clients' skin issues, like acne on the face and back, have completely disappeared since they've stopped consuming inflammatory foods such as dairy and processed pork. Several resolved their constipation and digestive disorders by removing gluten and wheat products. Others reduced their symptoms by abandoning alcohol.

Now that we recognize the difference between real foods and processed artificial foods, we can understand why certain methods, chemicals and additives in industrial food processing harm our bodies.

These foods irritate the lining of our gut and disrupt our natural detoxification pathways. They clog the body, promote mucus and cause inflammation, acne, brain fog and fatigue, amongst many other discomforts. They can also reduce muscle recovery.

Most of these foods are irritants to the body because they are either packed with chemicals or are genetically altered.

Cut the Crap Challenge – Triple C!

Experiment and experience for yourself: cut the crap for one to three weeks. Choose one item or choose 'em all. The beauty of cutting the crap is that there is always an alternative to substitute the crap you are cutting out. Check out my favourite Stable Table (page 159) for perfect delicious alternatives!

CCC Instructions:

1. Buy a notebook and title it "Triple C".

2. Check out the Stable Table and shop for healthier, less harmful and more sustainable alternatives to experiment with.

3. Choose one food category from the list above and remove it from your diet (gluten, for example) for one to three weeks.

4. Journal what you eat and pay attention to your mood, energy levels, how your stomach feels after eating, your digestion, and anything else you notice that changes for you.

At first you may feel empty or anxious, but distract yourself and eat plenty of alternatives to stay satisfied! To truly understand if your body is negatively affected, you must abstain from it for the one to three weeks, and when you reintroduce this food, eat it in the quantity you would have normally enjoyed. This way, you can understand if your body agrees with it or not.

NO FOOD IS FORBIDDEN, UNLESS THE BODY SAYS SO

Don't stress out. If you're a dairy lover, this doesn't mean that you can never consume cheese again, but it's a chance to discover which, if any, of these foods might be causing harm to your precious self. Don't just believe what I say, try for yourself, and learn from experience!

LETTING GO OF WHAT YOU LOVE WHEN IT'S TOXIC

Change can be scary and hard, but only for our minds. Our body loves positive change and it will thank you!

The mind (or ego) wants to hold on to comfortable old patterns.

To ease this process of change, I use the abundance approach. I dislike feeling hungry or deprived of joys in my life, especially when it comes to food. So I have never allowed myself nor my clients to feel restricted. Before we make any changes, we need to plan properly and fill our kitchen with abundant foods that will satisfy our mind – which is why the Love Real Food shopping lists are at the beginning of the book! (p. 63–5.) Focusing on the positive foods to eat, and making them exciting, delicious and fun, is key.

Jonathan's Story

"Danah and I went to school together when we were fourteen. I had really bad acne. I had tried everything. Danah suggested I try cutting out dairy. At that time, this was weird and unheard of. Milk was great! Although it sounded crazy, I tried to completely avoid dairy. Within two months, my acne was gone. My skin was super soft and glowing. I couldn't believe it!"

- Jonathan, age 30, cinematographer, San Diego

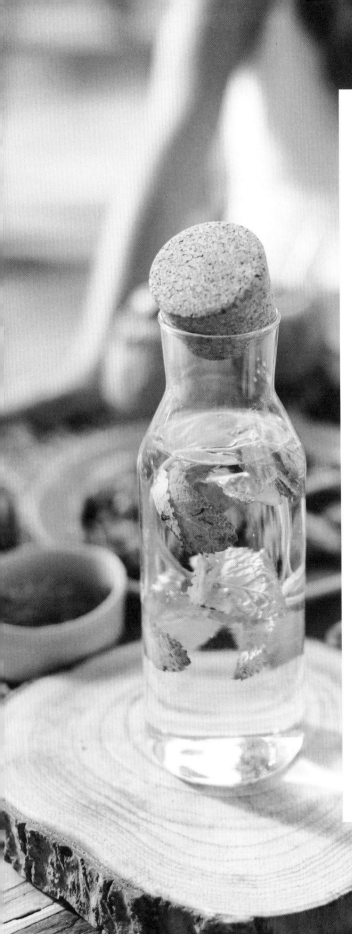

Daisy's Story

"When I removed gluten and dairy from my daily eating routine, my body felt light, energetic and happy. Bread and wheat-based cereals caused constipation, bloating and this constant feeling of fullness (which I strongly dislike!). Once I cut out gluten, I never felt that way again. Now that it's off the table, I can actually enjoy a pizza or sandwich once in a while without having the discomforts I had before. If I eat foods containing dairy or gluten for two or three days in a row, I start to feel the negative effects. Listening to my body helped me literally feel lighter in life with more energy and motivation to realize my objectives. My inner communication with my body is so much better that I can eat certain foods once in a while without the negative effects."

- Daisy, age 28, actress, London

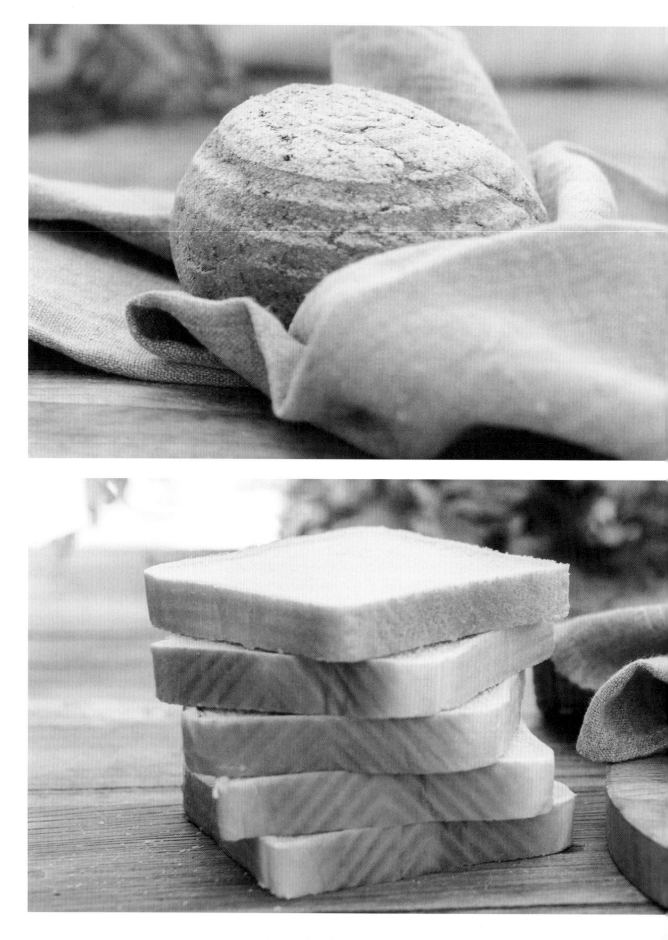

"Control your mind and your body will follow."

Ms Bihn, my seventh-grade English teacher

I now understand what she meant. The mind is very controlling and doesn't like change, no matter how good it feels to the body. The secret to making any change is to trick your mind so that it doesn't detect the change, and allow your body to follow. Your body is more flexible and adaptable than you think. Once the mental blockage is gone, you can truly understand the real effects of food on your body. Having rice or almond milk on your cereal, or rooibos tea with rice milk instead of black tea and cow's milk, are perfect examples of tricking your mind. Try it with your loved ones too. It's a great way to choose healthier, more sustainable foods without too much of a headache!

CROWDING OUT – THE SECRET

The only way cutting the crap stays fun is by crowding out. The secret to crowding out is substituting the "crap" with something similar but better. You can call it tricking your mind but, really, I think it's the opposite. You're finally getting a hold of it. This way, you're psychologically satisfied. There's no point depriving yourself of foods you're used to eating.

This is by far the most efficient trick in the book to making any change in your life. Finding ways to distract your mind as you take small steps toward a life you choose, rather than being a slave to your desires and cravings.

Check out the awesome Stable Table on page 159. This is a perfect way to make small changes at home that no one will notice. My clients love the Stable Table.

Daniela's story

"It's perfect to hang on the fridge. I use it when following ordinary recipes, using the good stuff to replace the crap. My boyfriend didn't notice the difference at first. Once he noticed (and I explained the health benefits), he actually preferred almond milk to dairy, and he loves quinoa instead of rice, and hummus instead of cheese!"

- Daniela, age 29

DAIRY

When we lived as farmers, milk was a nourishing food, rich in many enzymes, nutrients and fats. Now, milk and dairy production are multi-billion dollar industries. What has this done to the quality of the milk?

Milk has been sold to us for decades as a great source of calcium. This idea has become embedded in our culture.

I once gave a workshop on how the industrialization of food was changing the nature of food, and milk was brought up. One girl got really emotional in the discussion that followed my presentation. I later found out that her family were dairy farmers. It's hard to accept that a nourishing food like milk that sustains us as babies can be bad for us as adults; **just like with many foods, it's not the nature of the food, but how we have manipulated it to become an industrialized product.**

Science has now proven the hazardous health effects of cow's milk and other forms of dairy, from allergies to digestive disorders. Let's keep it simple and ask ourselves why we ever started drinking cow's milk in the first place. After all, drinking another species' milk is kinda strange if you think about it. Cow's milk is designed to turn a 35kg calf into a 200kg cow in twelve months! It's therefore very high in fat. The dairy industry takes this high-fat liquid, skims off the fat, and creates foods with an even higher fat content, such as butter, ice cream, yogurt and cheese. The consumption of these foods has been directly linked to chronic runny noses, sore throats, hoarseness, bronchitis, reoccurring ear infections, mucus from nose and throat, nausea, cramps, gas, bloating, diarrhoea, skin problems, acne and even heart disease, the number one killer of our society!

Technically, everyone is lactose-intolerant in varying degrees. We actually stop producing lactase, the enzyme that digests lactose, the sugar in milk, around age six.

So, why do we drink milk? Is it because it's so ingrained in our culture to do so? Is it because it's a good source of calcium? Do cows produce calcium or do they have to eat something rich in calcium so that their milk is rich in calcium too? How does this work and where does the calcium come from?

Let's say that cows do not produce calcium, therefore the calcium in cow's milk comes from the food that cows naturally eat.

We can all agree that a cow's natural diet is grass, which is super rich in calcium, as well as protein and numerous other nutrients. You could say that grass is a superfood. So, what happens when a cow no longer eats grass? Is her milk still rich in calcium? Unfortunately, the answer is no. That's why milk packaging nowadays often has the words "fortified with calcium" written on it. These products are injected with lab-produced artificial calcium which is very different from naturally occurring nutrients found in grass and real milk. So, modern milk is no longer rich in calcium, is highly processed and comes from unhappy cows lined up in factory farms, forced to produce milk non-stop for years on end, even milked when they are pregnant.

Did you know that calcium from animal milk is not as easily absorbed as calcium from plant-based sources?

DAIRY FARM REALITY

Our animals are no longer eating grass, or free to roam in the sun. They are confined to tiny enclosures where they are fed processed carbohydrate-rich food, which is low in vitamins, minerals and nutrients; they are injected with antibiotics to ensure they don't get sick, in order to increase production, reduce costs and grow profits.

"The milk we drink today is quite unlike the milk our ancestors were drinking, without apparent harm. The milk we drink today may not be nature's perfect food. Butter, meat, eggs, milk and cheese are implicated in hormone dependent cancers in general."
The Harvard Gazette

Many people have also chosen to ditch dairy because the hormones present in milk can be dangerous for human consumption. Some argue that the mistreatment of the animals conflicts with their ethical views, especially the practice of impregnating a cow solely for milk production, then removing its calf at birth, often to later slaughter it for veal.

If you really love dairy and want to continue consuming it, try reducing your consumption and find small local farmers who are producing dairy responsibly, on farms where the cows are happy, eating grass and free to roam outside.

WHEAT

Although we've been eating grains for ages, we've changed the way we eat them, especially wheat. First, we no longer eat them whole. As I explain in Love Real Food (p.36–65), we refine them and remove the best parts! Second, modern wheat is different to what our body is traditionally used to, and wheat's components are now causing allergies, inflammation and harm.

CUT WHEAT, CUT THE PROBLEM.

"The world's most popular grain is also the world's most destructive dietary ingredient."
William Davis, MD, author of Wheat Belly

A range of health issues has been linked to the consumption of wheat, from celiac disease, digestive and intestinal disorders, to neurological disorders and diabetes, heart disease, arthritis, rashes, even schizophrenia. If modern wheat

Sue's Story

My university nutrition professor, Sue, started out as a chef. She had a very frequent customer at her restaurant who had a wheelchair because of arthritis and joint pains. He moved away, but one summer, he walked back into the restaurant without his wheelchair. Sue asked him what had happened, how had he got rid of it? Her customer explained that he'd moved to Eastern Europe, where the wheat grains commonly used were not altered and genetically engineered, as he had been consuming in London. With the absence of modern wheat in his diet, his joint pain reduced and he slowly began walking again. Sue was so impressed by the curative power of food that she left her career as a chef and became a nutrition expert and professor.

is no longer what it used to be, perhaps we should consider other options. Chapter 4: Stock Up On Wholy Grains has a list of new alternatives to try, with cooking tips (p.74–83)! The Stable Table (p.159) also gives alternatives, which is useful if you are following a recipe.

GLUTEN - THE GLUE FACTOR

Wheat contains the protein gluten. Plants protect themselves by making their seeds poisonous so animals stay away. Wheat has a very short window for its seeds to grow and carry on the family line, so its seeds are more hostile than other grains.

Gluten is a protein found in grains like wheat, spelt, rye, kamut and barley. In Latin, "gluten" means "glue". If I eat gluten, I feel full and bloated all day. If I eat it for two consecutive days, I get constipated.

Gluten can stick to the intestinal wall and cause obstruction and inflammation. Imagine a papercut on your finger. That's how gluten irritates the lining of your gut, which then causes an inflammatory response. Gluten stimulates appetite by disrupting blood sugar levels, causing inflammation and aging.

Cutting out gluten has helped people eradicate chronic discomforts and unleash their natural energy levels and vitality. Others have reversed catastrophic health issues, including multiple sclerosis (MS), arthritis and ulcerative colitis. Try introducing naturally gluten-free grains (p.83) and check out the Stable Table for alternatives.

Lily's Story

When Lily first came to see me, she had suffered from chronic constipation since she was three years old. She said it was genetic, her siblings had the same problem. Lily went to the toilet once every two weeks - this was serious! I gave Lily two recommendations: 1. Morning ritual: Have a smoothie for breakfast after warm water with lemon. 2. Cut out gluten (wheat and other gluten-containing grains) completely for one week. Lily came to me three days later with the biggest smile on her face. She had already gone three times since she started the smoothie and cut out gluten. Lily goes to the toilet every day now!

SUGAR – MORE ADDICTIVE THAN COCAINE

Max's Story

"Let's be honest. I was an addict and sugar was my drug. However, after a morning of near complete shutdown in my early twenties, which induced a complete panic within me because of blood sugar woes, I, by chance, met a doctor who gave me some tips, which I followed very strictly for about six years. First, yes, you got it, NO sugar. It's everywhere in processed foods, so look carefully. Next, anything white and fluffy, just say no to as well. These foods convert to sugar very quickly and cause the spike and drop of blood sugar that affects so many of us. It was dramatically decreasing my quality of life. Hearing myself all the time saying, "I have to eat or I will die," and always saying no to long hikes unless I could pack food first was making me unhappy. So, I took a drastic step to help heal this problem within. No sugar, no white and fluffy stuff, I cut processed foods and meat consumption, and laid off alcohol. And voila! My body began to heal quite rapidly. Now I can enjoy a small slice of cake at someone's birthday, but in general, I still say no on almost all days of the year! And I am very happy to do so."

- Max, 35, wildlife expert, Connecticut, USA

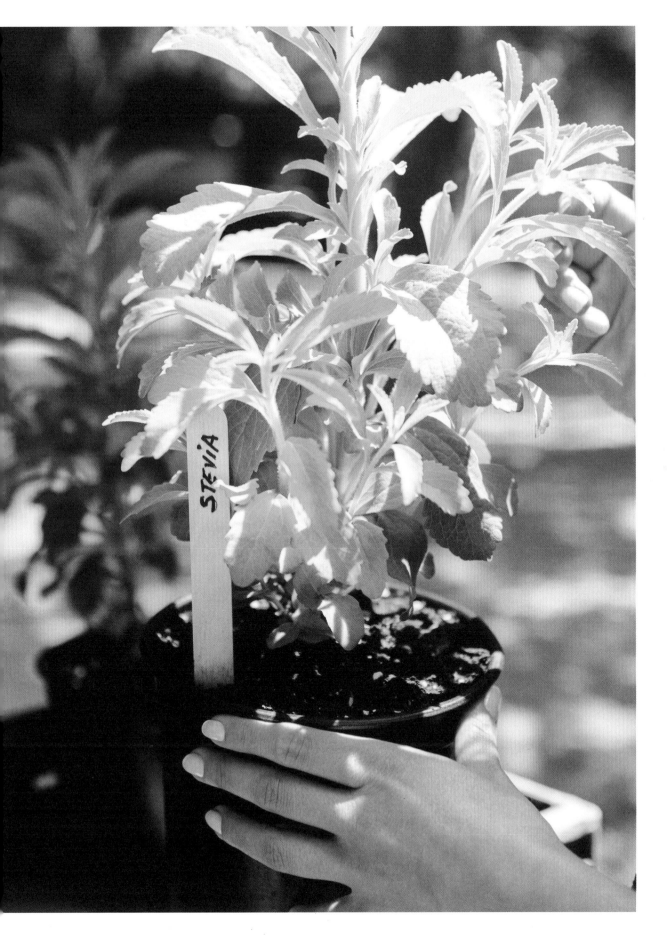

Sugar is added to almost everything nowadays. It is now considered the single worst ingredient in the modern diet. Sugar (glucose) is energy for all life forms, including our own cells. However, when we have more than our cells need, over time we lose the ability to control our blood sugar levels. This can lead to anxiety, depression, irritability, inflammation and weight gain, among many other issues. Sugar also feeds harmful microbes, bacteria, viruses and fungi. Which means we're likely feeding the cause of our discomfort with almost everything we eat. **Sugar is highly addictive, so it's really hard to cut out. It's also hidden almost everywhere!**

HERE ARE FIVE DISTURBING REASONS WE SHOULD CUT OUT SUGAR:

1. SUGAR IS NUTRIENT-LESS

Sugar contains lots of calories but zero nutrients. There are no proteins, essential fats, vitamins or minerals in sugar. Eating a lot of sugar at the expense of other foods has become a major contributor to nutrient deficiencies.

2. SIC: SUGAR, INSULIN AND CANCER

Too much sugar in our blood is highly toxic and dangerous, so the body produces a hormone called insulin that tells our cells to absorb sugar from the bloodstream, reducing levels in the blood. When we consistently consume a lot of sugary foods and drinks, we are causing our blood sugar levels to rise (which is dangerous), so the body keeps pumping out insulin to maintain a safe blood sugar level. The problem is that insulin regulates cell growth and has been seriously linked with cancer growth. Many scientists agree that constant elevated insulin levels (a consequence of chronic sugar consumption) contributes to cancer.

3. SUGAR FEEDS INFLAMMATION AND MAKES US FAT, SICK AND UNHAPPY

What sugar does to our body: Mix water with a few spoons of sugar and you'll get a syrup-like paste. Now, imagine your blood flowing around your body through its tiny vessels with this consistency. Flow is sticky, slow and ineffective. Tissues can become starved of oxygen, deteriorate, and die. Sugar can have harmful effects on metabolism and contributes to all sorts of diseases.

4. SUGAR CAUSES WRINKLES AND AGEING OF THE SKIN

This happens through glycation, which is where sugar attaches to a protein or lipid structure in the body. Glycation causes free radical damage, premature ageing and disease.

5. SUGAR IS MORE ADDICTIVE THAN COCAINE

Just like drugs such as cocaine, sugar causes a release of dopamine, the reward hormone, in the brain. Research published in the Public Library of Science highlights an experiment involving sugar and cocaine. Rats were given cocaine until they became dependent on it. Then researchers gave them a choice – the rats could continue to have the cocaine or they could switch to sugar. Guess which one the rodents chose? Yup, the sugar. A huge majority – 94 per cent – chose to make the switch. Even when they had to work harder to access the sugar, the rats were more interested in it than they were in the cocaine. Why? Because the sugar had a much more powerful effect on their brains. The same thing can be observed in humans.

How to Avoid Sugar

1. It's time to either read labels really well or just say no to processed foods. If sugar is one of the first three ingredients listed, put the product back on the shelf!

2. Make your own food, snacks, desserts and juices so you know what you're eating.

3. Enjoy your coffee and tea without sugar.

4. Choose real food with real flavours – this is how nature intended it – the best form of energy in the perfect dose.

5. Make sugar an occasional food, or forget it altogether. I've had a toxic relationship with sugar for a few years now. I find that lowering my dose works better than cutting it completely. Once I focus on other aspects in my life, my need to eat sugar vanishes. Others prefer to cut it out completely and avoid any foods that contain it, because it's so addictive. Find out what works for you!

REFINED CARBOHYDRATES

These include white flour and white pasta, and all other white fluffy foods. These foods do not taste sweet like sugar, but they do contain longer chains of sugars (starch). Refined carbohydrates are usually low in fibre too, as the high-fibre part has been removed. This means they cause blood sugar to spike more rapidly than non-refined wholefoods.

Refined grains are high-sugar, low-nutrient foods, while wholegrains are complex carbohydrates packed with nutrients along with the sugar in the middle of the grain. The fibre in the shell of the grain slows down the absorption of its sugars, which promotes healthy blood sugar levels. Always choose wholegrains and wholefoods.

PROCESSED FOODS

ARTIFICIAL SWEETENERS

I've always wanted to write a book called *Diet or Health, Choose One*, because they often mean opposite things. Food labelled with "diet" or "sugar-free" are often packed with additives, chemicals and artificial sweeteners, which may appear to be less fattening, but these substitutes are certainly more harmful.

Artificial sweeteners are chemically produced compounds that create a sweet flavour in food and drinks with no calories. They are 100 per cent chemical and artificial. Most people choose them over sugar for weight reasons, but it has been proven that these chemicals actually enhance your appetite and result in more weight gain than eating normal sugar. These fake sugar substitutes are up to **1,000 times sweeter** than normal sugar, so when you eat food with regular sugar, you actually need much more to satisfy your palate! That's crazy! Although some are considered safe, there hasn't been vigorous testing, so who really knows?

Artificial sweeteners are highly addictive. Especially when combined with caffeine, like in "diet" or "zero" drinks. Some research has shown that artificial sweeteners contain neurotoxins that attack brain cells and the nervous system. They have been linked to headaches, dizziness, mood swings, nausea, bowel complications, depression, anxiety, joint pain, arthritis, skin rashes, dementia and more. Argh!

Nowadays, there are more natural forms of zero calorie sweeteners, like stevia leaf, but beware of the highly processed forms you buy. The use of artificial sweeteners as a substitute for sugar is a controversial topic with conflicting research, and when I'm not sure, I choose natural and unprocessed. I prefer to enjoy the calories in real food!

Artificial sweeteners are hidden in chewing gum, sweets, drinks, "diet" and "zero" foods, pharmaceutical products, "sugar-free" foods and much more. If we stop buying the products, they may stop making them. Check your food for these fake forms of sugar and beware because the industry changes the names so we can't keep track:

* *Aspartame*
* *Acesulfame potassium*
* *Alitame*
* *Cyclamate*
* *Dulcin*
* *Equal*
* *Glucin*
* *Kaltame*
* *Mogrosides*
* *Neotame*
* *NutraSweet*
* *Nutrinova*
* *Phenlalanine*
* *Saccharin*
* *Splenda*
* *Sorbitol*
* *Sucralose*
* *Twinsweet*
* *Sweet'N Low*
* *Xylitol*

If you have to have sugar, choose natural sweeteners over artificial sweeteners, and when you're stronger, choose no sugar. Use cinnamon and other natural ingredients for sweetness and flavour. Check out the Love Real Food shopping list in Chapter 2 for alternatives.

BACKSTAGE: THE FOOD INDUSTRY AND WHAT'S INSIDE PROCESSED FOOD

During this last century, more than 3,000 food additives and chemicals have found their way into our food. When foods are packaged, canned, refined, puffed, dried, frozen and pre-cooked, they naturally

|153|

lose flavour, colour and visual appeal through food processing. So, manufacturers have to add chemicals to bring back the flavours and colours to make food look so good that we'll buy it. Just to give you an idea, adding additives like MSG restores flavour, while artificial colours and hydrogenated trans fats improve visual appearance. The sad thing is that these additives are toxic to our brains, our bodies, our moods, and our basic functions like digestion, thinking, learning, working and walking. Companies see opportunities in health trends and pretend to recreate "unhealthy" foods in a "healthy" way – like "diet" and "zero" drinks that are packed with "non-fattening" chemicals and artificial sweeteners. Other companies inject synthetic nutrients, colours and flavours and claim foods to be fresh, rich in vitamins and flavour.

All these processes make products easier to sell but worse for our bodies. They also make us think we can eat them more often. **If you're going to have a fizzy drink, have the original, with sugar and all. Just have it occasionally.** I've seen so many people drink diet cola every day because they think it's not making them fat or that it's not bad for them. This is exactly what the companies want us to do – blindly increase our consumption and their profits. They do not have our health or vitality in mind.

Most of the chemicals in processed foods have not been consumed by humans for very long, so we honestly don't know the extent of their effects on the body, which makes it best to avoid them. However, long-term studies are showing that toxic accumulation in the body causes cell mutation and eventually cancer. It's not a coincidence that these horrifying conditions have sky-rocketed since the boom of processed convenience foods.

These toxic substances are often hidden in processed foods, even healthy foods such as gluten-free bread. They are all harmful to the body, from disrupting our hormone function to reducing our immune responses, these new artificial substances are definitely not what we want to be feeding ourselves or our kids. Check ingredient labels and make a choice! All these additives have been scientifically considered carcinogenic in the body, they interfere with nutrient absorption, and can cause disease.

> "If you see any of these [artificial additives] on a food label, promptly put it back on the shelf; if you value your health, you don't want to be putting these in your body."
>
> *Andrea Donsky*

Label Reading

"Real food has no label." If we're going to buy food in a package with a label, let's start reading them. The tiny text is created so it's hard to read. Ingredients are listed in order of quantity, the first one being the main ingredient in the product. So, if you're buying apple juice and the first ingredient is sugar, then water, then apple, consider it sugar juice with apple flavour. You can apply this to all of your shopping. For example, almond butter should list almonds as its first ingredient, and so on. This simple exercise is super helpful when shopping as it cuts out the crap with little work.

PESTICIDES

The agriculture industry is a business, so sick crops mean less profits. The industry found ways to kill the bugs and pathogens that may harm crops. Pesticides are chemicals that are used to kill "pests" like insects, mice and other animals, weeds, fungi, bacteria, viruses and anything else that might try to destroy crops. If they are so harmful to living things, surely they are to us too?

Since the application of these chemicals is non-specific, other organisms are unintentionally exposed to them. The research shows that pesticides commonly harm, and kill, organisms other than pests, including humans. The World Health Organization estimates that there are three million cases of pesticide poisonings each year and up to 220,000 deaths.

Every year, more than one billion kilograms of pesticides are added to our food supply. Most of the pesticides used throughout the world are carcinogenic. Pesticide consumption and chemical accumulation has been linked to brain toxicity, hormone disruptions and cancer, a number of neurological problems including memory loss and mood swings, allergies, hypersensitivity, infertility and foetal developmental problems, amongst other common disorders.

> *"The chemical for bombs was altered to make pesticide, another was tweaked to become herbicide and sprayed onto all of our vegetables."*
> *Paul Connett, PhD*

After World War I, there were huge amounts of toxic chemicals left over. Instead of disposing of them, it was decided it would be a profitable option to sell these toxic chemicals to farmers.

How does this make sense? We are being sold foods that are sprayed with chemicals that have been used to kill humans.

How harmful these pesticides are to our bodies and organs on a cellular level is being understood today through more reports and studies that link human disease to pesticide consumption.

Several pesticides that were once considered safe are now banned. This shows us that newly invented chemicals are difficult to consider safe and are often launched into our food supply without proper proof of safety, and only banned once they are proven unsafe by consumers (through effective poisoning). Basically, WE are paying to test a product with our own money and health.

Some of the worst chemicals known to man are put into our foods. Roundup, a very commonly used pesticide, is now considered to be a carcinogen. This is only one of many examples.

PESTICIDE FACTS
Pesticides:
* *Contaminate our water systems, our fresh water rivers and lakes.*
* *Destroy and intoxicate gardens that are downstream from sprayed fields.*
* *Pollute our air.*
* *Infect our food.*
* *Harm our organs and cells: just like they kill bacteria and insects, they are slowly destroying us.*

If pesticides were labelled on vegetables and foods, it would offer us an informed choice. Unfortunately, we are kept ignorant

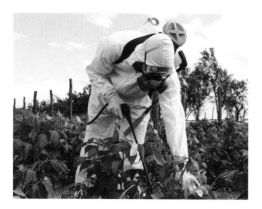

for clear reasons. Perhaps we could be asking if the increase of toxic chemicals in our food, clothes and water is one of the reasons for the increase in childhood disease, especially cancer.

Strawberries are highly sprayed. Because they have very thin skin, they absorb most of the chemicals sprayed on them and cause many allergies. Think of how many kids love strawberries! Buy them organic!

If you don't make these choices for yourself, make them for the planet and for your children.

HOW TO REDUCE YOUR PESTICIDE EXPOSURE

Because pesticides don't die or biodegrade, they are washed into our water supply, travel in the air, and stay on the fruits and veggies we eat. They are literally everywhere. Since we can't avoid them completely, it's useful to know how to reduce your absorption of pesticides to a minimum.

Filtering your drinking water and opting for organic produce whenever possible will dramatically reduce your exposure to pesticides. The Dirty Dozen and Clean Fifteen (see overleaf) are helpful lists developed by our friends at the Environmental Working Group that help us to understand which fruits and vegetables are most and least contaminated by pesticides respectively. These lists are great when it comes to budgeting for organic fruit and veg. Always try to get the veggies on the Dirty Dozen list organic. These foods have thin skin and easily absorb the chemicals sprayed onto them.

On the other hand, the Clean Fifteen are veggies and fruits that have thicker skin and don't easily absorb the sprayed chemicals. Nevertheless, if you can't buy the dirty dozen organic, don't start avoiding them altogether. Veggies are always packed with nutrients that will make you strong and happy either way! Also, get to know your farmers, ask them what they use to protect their crops. Become informed about what goes into your mouth. No pesticides are good for the environment, nature, wildlife or our water systems, so preventing them is only positive!

ORGANIC PRODUCE

Buying organic whenever possible is not only better for your health and reduces your exposure to GMO foods and pesticides, but it also sends a message that you support environmentally friendly farming practices that minimize soil erosion, protect employees and protect water quality, wildlife and nature.

The benefits of eating conventionally grown vegetables and greens exceeds the negative effects of pesticides. So, ALWAYS opt for conventionally grown veggies when organic is not an option instead of skipping them. Don't avoid the dirty dozen if you can't buy them organic. They are still fresh vegetables packed with goodness. Be fuelled by veggies!

Organic foods can be more costly, so get down with the Dirty Dozen and the Clean Fifteen to help prioritize what veggies and fruits to invest in!

SO, Cutting the Crap is about understanding what foods actually harm our bodies and taking them out of our day-to-day eating habits as much as possible. I ditched these foods a long time ago, which means I no longer shop for them and keep them out of my house. Every once in a while, I can still enjoy a real French croissant! Being aware that these foods interfere with the proper functioning of the body, and make us tired, slow and puffy, makes it easier for us to consume less of them and find a balance. And if you have them, notice how you feel, and make sure your indulgence is occasional. Embrace this chapter with common sense and moderation. What you do every day is important, not once in a while. Voila!

THE DIRTY DOZEN
Get these organic when possible!

Apples
Celery
Sweet bell peppers
Peaches
Strawberries
Nectarines
Grapes
Spinach
Lettuce
Cucumbers
Blueberries
Potatoes
Also, green beans and kale are moving up on the most sprayed list as well.

CLEAN FIFTEEN
These aren't sprayed as heavily, so buy non-organic if you're budgeting.

Onions
Avocado
Sweet Corn (GMO)
Pineapple
Mango
Sweet Peas
Aubergine/Eggplant
Cauliflower
Asparagus
Kiwi
Cabbage
Watermelon
Grapefruit
Sweet Potatoes
Honeydew Melon

STABLE TABLE
Experiment and use this table to re-build ordinary recipes

CURRENT INGREDIENT	ALKALINE INGREDIENT
Milk	Plant-based milk (except for soy) *read the ingredients to make sure soy isn't included
Meat	Beans, grains and vegetables
Mince	Black beans or red rice burgers
Cheese (in a sandwich or wrap)	Hummus, avocado/guacamole, grilled vegetables, baba ganoush
Boxed Breakfast Cereals	Gluten-free oat flakes with raisins, banana slices and plant-based milk, gluten-free granola with plant milk
Pasta	Wholegrain, gluten-free pasta
White Rice	Brown basmati, quinoa, millet or red rice
Potatoes	Sweet potato
Sugar	Stevia leaf, coconut sugar, ground cinnamon
Butter/Margarine	Coconut oil, avocado slice, olive oil
Salad Dressing	Lemon juice, olive oil (plain or with tahini)
Vinegar	Lemon juice, umeboshi plum vinegar (sometimes)
Tomato Sauce/ketchup	Blended fresh tomato, olive oil and garlic
Coffee/Black Tea	Rooibos tea with plant-based milk
Frying Oil	Steam-fry or use coconut oil
Pizza	Rice/corn make good pizza dough. Add mushrooms, onions, garlic, olives, fresh herbs for toppings
Chips	Slow-baked sprouted breads, gluten-free wraps, sliced sweet potatoes, beetroot (beets) with herbs and salt
Standard Bread	Freshly baked gluten-free bread, sprouted breads
Mayonnaise	Hummus or guacamole
Yogurt	Coconut yogurt, sweet smoothies such as banana, almond butter and almond milk
Table Salt	Himalayan salt, *fleur de sel*

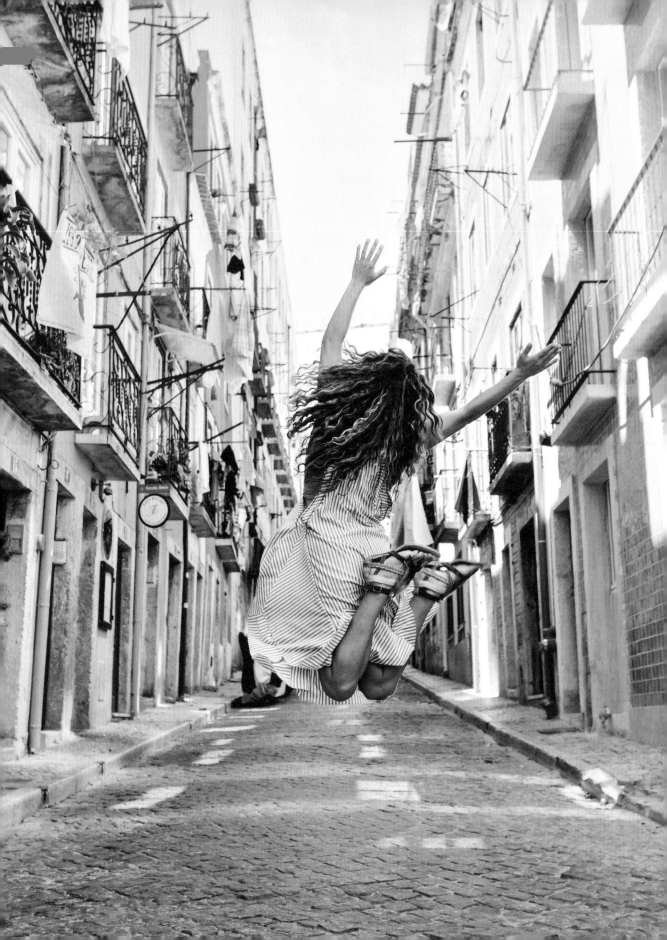

> *"We humans have become the most chemically contaminated species on the planet."*
>
> *Dr Brian Clement, PhD, Hippocrates Health Institute*

Chapter 9

TAKE OUT THE TRASH EVERY DAY (TOTE)

DETOXIFY DAILY

THIS IS MY FAVOURITE CHAPTER, BECAUSE LIFE DRASTICALLY CHANGES WHEN YOUR BODY CAN FINALLY RID ITSELF OF THE LETHAL WASTE AND TOXINS IT HAS ACCUMULATED OVER TIME.

LEARN HOW TO INCORPORATE DAILY DETOX INTO YOUR EVERYDAY HABITS TO BOOST YOUR MOOD, ENERGY AND BRAIN POWER. YOU WILL NOTICE LESS IRRITATION, FATIGUE AND FOGGY THINKING, MORE RESISTANCE, ENERGY AND FOCUS. YOU WON'T KNOW WHAT HIT YOU.

From air pollution, cleaning detergents and body care products, to petrochemicals in our modern clothing, medications, birth control pills, synthetic supplements, alcohol, processed foods, pesticides and polluted water, we inhale, ingest and absorb toxins all the time. They are everywhere.

On an individual level, there are two things that will help our body and planet reduce this toxic overload. **First**, reduce toxic exposure whenever and wherever possible. **Second**, unblock and stimulate the existing pathways that eliminate toxins from our bodies every day. This is the TOTE concept.

Just like in our home, we need to take our trash out every day. We need to continuously stimulate our natural pathways for eliminating toxins. If we create a rhythm of daily elimination, we avoid toxic accumulation and overload, protecting our bodies. Toxicity causes inflammation and the perfect environment for dysfunction and disease.

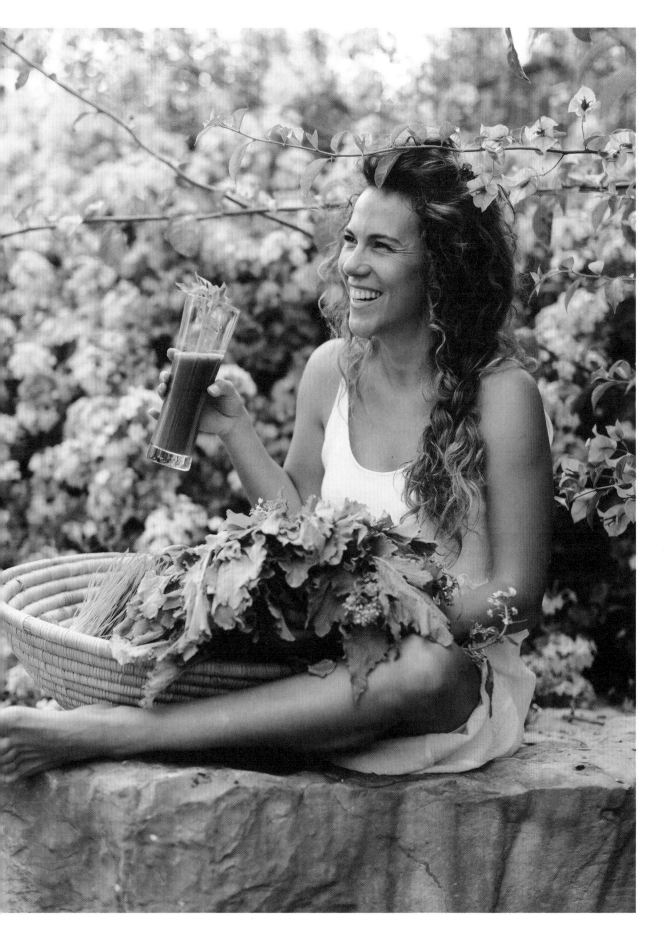

DETOX YOUR BODY: FROM TOXIC BUILD-UP TO OVERLOAD

Is ignorance bliss? What we don't know doesn't hurt us, right? Wrong. The catch is that what you don't know, you can't change, and so it will eventually cause you harm. Toxins can stay in our body and accumulate over days, months, even years! Most of us carry toxins from several years ago, which cause lethargy, fatigue, brain fog, allergies, irritation, mood swings and more serious conditions like autoimmune disorders, heart disease and cancer. If your liver is congested and you continue to feed yourself more toxicity, what do you think might happen?

Toxins interfere with normal body functioning, confusing our normal bodily processes and causing stress to our internal environment.

By Loving Real Food and Cutting The Crap, we minimize inflammatory foods in our diet that cause toxic accumulation and eventually clog our elimination pathways that work so hard to keep us strong and healthy! This instantly improves the way we feel every day because our body is able to rid itself of daily waste. However, food isn't the only thing influencing toxicity.

Here are examples of non-foods that increase toxic accumulation in the body:

* Stress
* Pollution
* Synthetic chemicals (detergents, clothes, medication)
* Lack of sleep
* Negative emotions/thoughts

Stress is definitely my biggest toxic enemy. Finding ways to de-stress are crucial to my vitality. Creative forms of expression like playing an instrument, dancing or light physical movement have helped me and many of my clients relax, and get out of their head, which allows for relaxation. I started playing the piano again recently and found that tapping into my creativity really helped me connect with my body and to de-stress.

Further into the chapter we take it to the next step by finding ways to reduce toxicity at home – one of the main places we spend time in that we can actually change!

Once we have that organized, Chapter 13 *You are What you ~~Eat~~ Think* takes detoxing to the deepest level. Here we start to become aware of our thoughts and inner conversations and how they can positively or negatively affect us.

THE LIVER, MY FAVOURITE ORGAN

The liver is the body's number one cleansing organ. As the second largest organ in the body (after the skin), one of its functions is neutralizing toxins from everything we eat, drink, breathe and apply onto our skin.

When the liver functions well, we feel good, have consistent energy, proper hormone balance, good sleep, good moods and clear skin. Life is good, and we are a joy!

Weight gain, irritability, fatigue, feeling puffy or inflamed, acne, skin rashes, joint pain, high cholesterol, depression, brain fog and irritability can simply be signs of an overworked or congested liver.

All toxins have to be detoxed by the liver. The body is perfectly built to eliminate toxins all day, every day, through its **detoxing pathways**:

sweating, breathing, urinating, bowel movements and lymph drainage.

That's why it's super important that we drink enough water, evacuate our bowels every day, sweat enough, and don't block our skin pores with synthetic/plastic clothing.

Our skin eliminates toxins. Wear natural fibres or don't wear clothes at all!

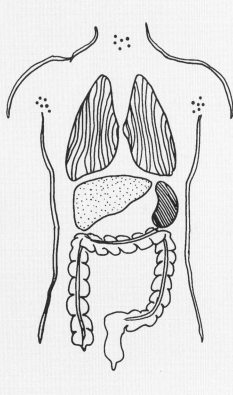

Major detoxing organs: skin, liver, lungs, kidneys, large intestines and lymphatic system (largest filter system in the body).

|165|

GLOWING SKIN AND LYMPH

We don't talk much about our lymph system, although we may have heard of lymphatic drainage massage. Our lymph is the biggest filtering system in the body. It's a circulatory system, like blood, and its functions are like a vacuum cleaner, transporting toxins and waste products out of the body. While the heart pumps blood around, our lymph system has no pump at all. Its circulation depends completely on our movement and physical activity. The contractions of our muscles keep our lymph moving and eliminate the toxicity it gathers from all around the body. Our lymph system lies just below the skin, influencing its brightness. Glowing skin is the result of a healthy lymph system that keeps moving. Our lymph likes gentle movement and exercise like stretching, walking, swimming or yoga. So what are you waiting for? Get gently moving!

BREAKING THE FAST: DEMYSTIFYING THE BREAKFAST HYPE

Your morning routine is key to setting the tone for the day. What you do or eat in the morning will influence your dietary choices for the rest of the day. Breakfast is literally breaking a fast. During the night, your organs begin to cleanse and detox. However, most of us cut this process short by stuffing ourselves with heavy solid foods in the morning. When we prolong the detox process, the body has longer to be in "cleanse" mode and expel toxins before it has to focus again on digestion. Toxic elimination takes place on several layers, like an onion. By encouraging and prolonging our natural detox processes whenever possible, we are encouraging deeper forms of toxic elimination, including organ and cellular cleansing.

It's not natural to eat straight away when you wake up. As hunters and gatherers we had to go out each morning and find our food. We didn't have a fridge filled with high-sugar foods ready and waiting for us to eat. In fact, we often had to walk, move and exercise before consuming any calories. By nature, it is normal to allow time after awaking before we eat. Naturally this also enhances our cleansing process on a daily basis. When you wake up in the morning, drink water and fluids, allowing the body to regenerate itself slowly before you bring all the attention to your digestive tract; after all, our body only cleanses when we stop eating food.

If toxic elimination is more complete, digestion is enhanced and more nutrients can be absorbed from the food we eat.

The best way to break a fast is to drink. Drink water or drink highly nutritious juice, like a freshly pressed chlorophyll-rich green juice. This juice being pure liquid doesn't simply hydrate the body, but also replenishes nutrient levels, which directly boosts the cleansing process as it stimulates and improves our detox pathways. This high-nutrient (low-sugar) alkalizing green juice will satisfy your habit for food, which again will allow your body to prolong and continue your detox process! It's a win-win situation!

Intermittent fasting

This is a form of intermittent fasting. If you already practise intermittent fasting, pure green vegetable juice doesn't interfere with insulin production, and is therefore a perfect nutrient-rich food that doesn't break your fasting.

Pure vegetable (fruitless) green juices are suitable to ingest during the fast stage of intermittent fasting as they do not interfere with our blood sugar levels.

THE BENEFITS OF VEGETABLE GREEN JUICE

Benefits of daily detoxing and breaking the fast with liquids (a.k.a. juicing for breakfast):
* *Reduces cravings throughout the day by balancing blood sugar*
* *Stable/consistent energy*
* *Stronger immune system*
* *Mental clarity*
* *Clears sinuses*
* *Deeper sleep*
* *Less bloating*
* *Slimmer body*
* *Healthy sex drive*
* *Glowing skin*
* *Less inflammation*
* *Increased longevity*
* *Sparkling eyes*
* *Strong hair and nails*
* *Daily bowel movements*
* *Happy organs*
* *Lowered blood pressure (without medication)*
* *Lowered cholesterol*
* *Healthier joints*
* *Stronger bones*
* *Prevents depression*
* *Feeling of joy for no reason*

|167|

15 Tips for TOTE

Helping your body eliminate toxins daily can drastically improve your mood and life! Support your body and liver on a daily basis by introducing these everyday cleansing practices.

1. **Drink warm lemon water.** Hydrate first thing in morning. Start the day with a glass of warm water with some fresh lemon juice and a pinch of cayenne pepper. No matter where you are or what you do, you can always get your hands on a big glass of water, and if you're lucky, a lemon to squeeze into it. This alone will stimulate and prolong toxin elimination for your entire system. Lemon stimulates your liver and digestive functioning and cayenne pepper ignites and cleanses your circulatory system.

2. **Drink your breakfast.** Extend the cleansing process by having a cold-pressed juice on an empty stomach (or a wheatgrass shot). This way, your body absorbs the nutrients immediately. Don't automatically jump to solid food. Instead, wait until your body signals hunger. Have a green juice or smoothie as your first meal of the day. Drink it until full. Increase the size of your smoothie so that it becomes your only food until lunch. My daily choice is my green juice or, if I'm hungry, the Mean Green Smoothie. See p.187 for the recipes!

3. **Breathe fresh air.** Walk outside. Open windows. Breathe deeply!

4. **Jump.** Rebounding stimulates your lymphatic system and increases circulation. Twenty minutes of rebounding has the same benefits as a three-hour lymphatic massage.

5. **Sweat.** Sweating eliminates toxins and is one of the main ways the body eliminates acids. Sit in a sauna (infrared is best) and exercise with extra layers to increase perspiration and toxin elimination.

6. **Dance every day.** Exercise is the best way to enhance circulation, which stimulates organ and cellular detoxification. Our lymph is our internal vacuum cleaner, absorbing toxins and waste. The only way the lymph can circulate and eliminate toxicity is through mild physical activity. Dancing also helps de-stress!

7. **Dry body brush.** Before showering, take two minutes to dry brush your body from toes to neck to stimulate the lymphatic system. Softly brush your skin with a dry hand towel or exfoliating brush using long strides toward the heart.

8. **Eat probiotic enzyme-rich food,** like fermented foods that support digestion, nutrient absorption and regulate bowel movements.

9. **Get deep sleep.** When we're sleeping, our bodies are working hard to repair and recharge our vital organs and detox pathways. Depriving ourselves of sleep can interfere with natural detoxification pathways as well as affect our heart and the cardiovascular system.

10. **Eat enough fibre.** Fibre-rich foods bind up toxins in your intestines and keep your visits to the toilet regular. Constipation can cause reabsorption of toxins in your gut.

11. **Make your home experience the best.** Use natural cleaning products, have plants, and open windows! See the section on pages 170–178 on detoxing your home to take this further.

12. **Wear natural clothing.** Choose fibres that allow the skin to breathe and eliminate toxins, such as cotton, linen, silk or wool – or best of all, wear none at all!

13. **Use natural cosmetics.** Check out the Skin Deep website to see the ratings of body care products. Avoid products with the word "fragrance" or "parfum" in their ingredient list as they are endocrine disrupters. They interfere with our hormones, which make up the communication system of our entire body. These disruptors create miscommunication, causing us to perhaps feel hungry when we should feel sleepy, tired when we should feel awake, or confused when it's time to focus.

14. **Scrape your tongue.** Remove accumulated bacteria and toxic debris from the day and night before from your tongue. This will also improve your breath.

15. **Detox your mind of negative thoughts and chatter.** Only allow space for positive thoughts, as thoughts become chemistry in our body.

DETOX YOUR HOME: TAKE IT TO THE NEXT LEVEL

"Grant me the serenity to accept the things I cannot change, courage to change the things I can, and wisdom to know the difference."

Serenity Prayer, Reinhold Niebuhr

Detoxing daily is having the wisdom to know that you can change and then the courage to do it.

When we talk about toxicity, we usually think we can't change much. We can't change the air we breathe, the cars on the road, the tap water contaminants... but are there changes that we CAN make? Do we have the courage to change what we can control, like what we buy, what goes inside of our bodies, into our homes, and into the trash?

Did You Know?

The most polluted air environment is found inside of our homes. Studies show that most homes have the lowest concentration of oxygen at 6 per cent, lower than a polluted city!

Oxygen levels:
In a forest: 21 per cent
In a city: 11 per cent
Inside the house: 6 per cent

Every single environmental agency says that **the inside air is six to seven times more polluted than outside.** This is because of what we buy and put inside our homes, work spaces and schools.

We've concentrated on detoxifying our internal homes – our bodies. Now it's time to detox our external home. Home is a place where we can control the environment and make improvements to reduce and avoid toxicity for our

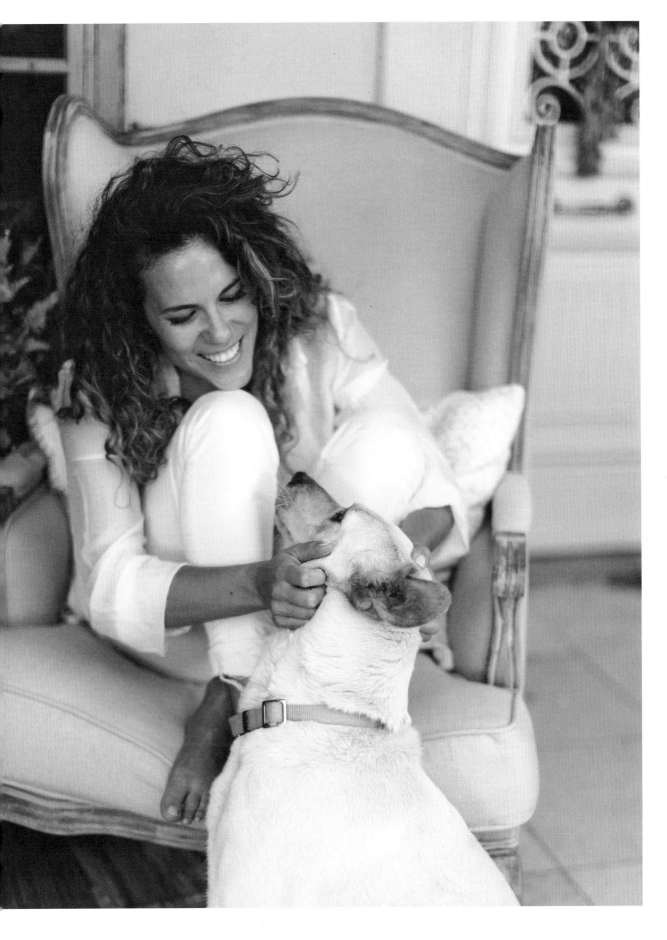

bodies and the planet. **Keeping our home environment friendly, safe and healthy is fundamental.**

PETROCHEMICALS

With advances in technology, new fabrics have been created that are all basically made of petrol. As petroleum is highly flammable, these fabrics undergo toxic treatments to adapt them – all because it's cheaper than using cotton and natural products. So when buying clothes or bed linen, or choosing a new sofa, carpet or curtains, make sure you check the labels and choose natural – especially for clothes that are in contact with your skin and all fabrics at home!

How much petrol is in your home?

Petroleum, the dangerous substance we all fuel our cars with, is used in many products we have in our homes today. The only thing is, we don't know that we are surrounded by it, and it's slowly polluting our home environment!

All petroleum-derived products have a harmful impact on human health and the ecosystem.

* *The toxicity of petroleum-related products threatens human health and the ecosystem. Many substances found in oil are highly toxic and carcinogenic. Oil emulsions in the digestive systems of many mammals can result in decreased ability to digest nutrients, and this can lead to their death.*
* *Other symptoms include capillary ruptures and haemorrhages.*
* *Ecosystem food chains can be affected due to a decrease in algae productivity, threatening several species.*
* *Oil is "acutely lethal" to fish – that means it kills fish quickly.*

Since manufacturers and governments don't seem to mind, it is our responsibility to ensure we reduce our absorption and exposure as much as possible – especially in our homes, where we can control the environment!

IS YOUR SOFA SLOWLY POISONING YOU?

Thousands of household products like synthetic fabrics, carpets, paints and cleaning products emit VOCs (volatile organic compounds), which are gases that damage the environment and our indoor air, which have serious adverse effects on our short- and long-term health. This is what makes our indoor air so much more toxic than the outside air.

At room temperature these

molecules in the products we buy evaporate into the air that we breathe! This means that our synthetic carpets and furniture, and our cleaning products, are slowly having a toxic effect on us.

Petrochemicals are any products derived from petroleum or petrol – one of the most dangerous liquids we know! These synthetic petrol-derived chemicals are so versatile that they are used in thousands of products we use daily – from being added into our food (which is toxic) and our self-care products (which is also toxic) to making car pieces and rocket fuel. Petrochemicals are also used to make plastics, fibres and synthetic rubber, and so if we're not careful we find them in almost all household products, including:

* Carpeting
* Detergents
* Perfume
* Shampoo
* Facial creams
* Deodorants
* Soft contact lenses
* Fertilizers
* Milk jugs
* Wax
* Crayons

Petrochemicals are pretty much everywhere – it's hard to avoid them completely. BUT, we can definitely reduce our absorption of petroleum by avoiding certain substances in all our household and selfcare products – all of which are absorbed through our skin. Dr Epstein, toxicologist and founder of the Cancer Prevention Coalition, found that many of the ingredients used in personal care and household products are industrial chemicals, including carcinogens, pesticides, reproductive toxins and hormone disruptors. Many of these products include highly toxic chemicals used in paint to keep it smooth (surfactants), soft concrete and other industrial methods we can recognize as being highly dangerous. **We are unknowingly putting these chemical toxins onto our skin and into our homes.**

|173|

TOXIC BEAUTY

Audit your self-care and cleaning products and ensure they don't contain any of the following toxic petrochemicals.

* BHA and BHT
* Benzene
* DEA-related ingredients – anything with DEA (diethanolamine) or MEA (ethanolamine)
* PEG (polyethylene glycol) related ingredients
* Anything ending in "eth" indicates that it required ethylene oxide (a petrochemical) to produce e.g. myreth, oleth, laureth, ceteareth
* Butanol and any word with "butyl" – butyl alcohol, butylparaben, butylene glycol
* Ethanol and any word with "ethyl" – ethylalcohol, ethylene glycol, ethylene dichloride, EDTA (ethylene-diamine-tetracetatic acid), ethylhexylglycerin
* Any word with "propyl" – isopropyl alcohol, propylene glycol, propyl alcohol, cocamidopropyl betaine
* Methanol and any word with "methyl" – methylalcohol, methylparaben, methylcellulose
* XParfum or fragrance – 95 per cent of chemicals used in fragrance are from petroleum
* Coal tar dyes: p-phenylenediamine and colours listed as "CI" followed by a five digit number
* Formaldehyde-releasing preservatives
* Parabens
* Siloxanes
* Sodium laureth sulfate
* Triclosan (a carcinogenic pesticide used in deodorants and much more)
* Paraffin wax

Most of these chemicals are harmful to our health and to the environment as they wash down our drain and damage or kill our wildlife!

CLEANING PRODUCTS

Anything that is toxic will evaporate into the air and be absorbed by you, your babies or pets – so when it comes to cleaning materials, keep it natural and clean. Avoid products that contain ammonia, DEA, APE, and TEA. Choose biodegradable detergents that decompose in nature and don't destroy our oceans and environment. If these products cost too much, I use good ol' wine vinegar, one of the best household cleaners. It's non-toxic and super low-cost. **Vinegar kills more microbes than most detergents do.** Use hot water and vinegar for floors, counter tops and windows. Don't worry, the smell disappears shortly after!

TOXIC CLOTHES

"Every product sold on the market that touches our skin is a test of our sensitivity because the chemical ingredients in the product are usually untested for their impact on human health before marketing occurs, which makes us all guinea pigs in an uncontrolled experiment."

Brian Clement PhD, Author of Killer Clothes

Nowadays, many clothes are made from synthetic fibres, usually nylon, acrylic, polyester and polypropylene. These are made from non-renewable petroleum and emit harmful volatile organic compounds (VOCs) into the air. VOCs easily become vapour or gas, most of which are dangerous air pollutants. When we wear them our body also absorbs these toxic chemicals.

Toxic fabrics to avoid in clothing:
Especially those in contact with your skin!
* *Polyester*
* *Nylon*
* *Acrylic*
* *Poly- anything (petro)*
* *Rayon*

Acetate and Triacetate. These are made from wood fibres called cellulose. However, they undergo extensive chemical processing to produce the finished product.

Instead choose these natural fibres:
* *Cotton*
* *Silk*
* *Linen*
* *Hemp*
* *Wool*
* *Cashmere*
* *Bamboo*

|175|

FURNITURE AND FABRIC

Similarly, when it comes to furniture and textiles, stick to natural options, like cotton and linen bedding, curtains and carpets. Choose wood where possible, especially for flooring. All petro-textiles are packed with more than a few chemicals, like stain-resistant treatments, anti-static chemicals and flame retardants, which are known to cause poor brain development, learning memory deficiencies and behavioural problems in children. Not to mention they are carcinogenic. These synthetic fabrics have VOCs that evaporate into the air, polluting your home environment and your body as they are inhaled! Choose fibres that don't contain:

* Flame-retardant chemicals
* Stain-guard or water-repellant finishes
* Antistatic chemicals

To protect furniture from spills and pets, choose a natural washable cover instead! All my curtains, carpets, bedding and sofa covers are cotton or linen and very washable.

EVERYTHING YOU DO MATTERS

When you live in a city, you don't see how the chemicals you use affect nature.

"When I was young, our kitchen sink water flowed right into the garden where a flush of plants and flowers grew abundantly from this "waste" water. When more modern detergents came out, I remember that the green plants and flowers disappeared – they had all died."

Dr Anna Maria Clement, Hippocrates Health Institute

The chemicals in modern household detergents destroy nature. Our "waste" water flows into rivers, lakes, seas and oceans. These chemicals do not biodegrade; they enter our water system and re-enter our homes in our own tap water. The umbilical cords of new-born babies have been found to contain more than 200 different chemicals before they are even born! This is passed to them through mama's exposure to the world. Be the example and start using smarter cleaning, decorating and beauty products.

Tips for Home Detoxing

1. **Keep your home air environment clean and oxygen-rich.** Open windows, have plants and avoid synthetic carpets, couch lining, curtains etc. Petro materials release chemicals into the air.

2. **Buy natural clothing, including cotton, linen, silk and wool.** Avoid 100 per cent polyester, nylon and other petrochemicals.

3. **Choose natural herbal remedies when possible.** Avoid any medications where possible, and synthetic supplements. Read ingredient lists, as companies are allowed to write "natural" on their packages when they use 90 per cent chemical ingredients. The law only requires a product to contain 10 per cent natural ingredients in order for it to be able to be labelled natural. This is crazy!

4. **Choose organic, biodegradable and natural household detergents.** They don't have to be more expensive; vinegar is the best and cheapest cleaner. Its strong smell disappears after minutes. **Vinegar kills more microbes than most detergents do.**

5. **Avoid aluminum.** It is found in deodorants, antacids and cookware.

6. Choose fragrance-free, paraben-free, fluoride-free body care products. General rule for skin products: **If you can't eat it, don't put it on your skin.**

7. **Buy organic food when possible.** Check out the Dirty Dozen and Clean Fifteen shopping guides on page 158.

8. **Filter your water of chlorine, fluoride and other contaminants.**

9. **Reduce electromagnetic stress.** Shut off your Wi-Fi router at night. Buy plugs/extension cords with on/off switches. Keep the base of a cordless phone far from your bed or not at all.

10. **Invest in real foods.** Avoid processed, chemical-packed foods.

YOUR TRASH - ZERO WASTE

We can't change the air we breathe. Or can we? Did you know that the plastic you throw away in the trash is burned and becomes the air you breathe? So, in the end, we can affect the air we breathe.

What happens to most of the waste we throw away every day? It gets burned or buried. Either way, chemicals in plastic are not biodegradable, meaning they cannot be broken down, and therefore cause harm to the environment in so many different ways. The synthetic, artificial molecules and chemicals in plastic, pharmaceuticals, pesticides, household detergents and cosmetics that are not biodegradable stay intact forever – this means they do not decompose to become part of a plant or a cell in our body. **When something is not made in nature it can never become part of nature.** These tiny particles intoxicate us as they flow through our water, air and food systems. When they're burned, they evaporate into the air and we then breathe them in; when they're buried, they are absorbed by the earth and get into our water and food systems. Either way, they get back to us.

Fish have been found to contain thousands of particles of plastic that are too small to see but we eat these particles when we eat the fish. Not to mention, fish themselves die if they become overloaded with these plastics.

So, reducing the amount of waste we throw into the garbage and down the toilet or sink can really make a difference to the quality of our water, air and soil. Here are a few ways to reduce our waste and protect our wildlife, our planet and our vitality!

1. Reduce: Reduce the amount you buy or use in the first place.

2. Reuse: Before you throw anything away, think about how you might be able to re-use it instead of buying something new.

3. Recycle: Although recycling is a good thing, it still requires a lot of energy to create a new product. If we can reduce the number of things we make or use in the first place, we are avoiding all forms of pollution created in recycling production, packaging and transportation. Reusing avoids the pollution involved in recycling while recycling avoids depleting our natural sources.

4. Start composting: Separate your organic trash from paper, plastic and glass. Find out if there is a composting ground near you, a farm, a family garden, etc. This bypasses any process and gets the nutrients back into the soil immediately. I compost in my back garden and keep it strictly vegetarian (no bones or meat) so rats and other fun animals stay away. Colourless paper and cardboard are also good for composting!

A WORD ON POO

You can change your life by looking backwards.

As uncomfortable as it may be to talk about, it's an ancient belief that the quality of your stools reflects the quality of your health. So, here's a little 101 on poo and keeping it regular.

COLON HEALTH, IMMUNITY, POOING AND ALL THAT JAZZ

Our gut is the control centre of our vitality, our "second brain". In fact, 70 per cent of our immune system lives in our gut. So, yes, we should be talking about our bowel movements more often.

At health school in Florida, we all arrived on day one, naturally embarrassed to talk about our poo. By day five, our embarrassment no longer existed. It was the talk of the day, always the first thing we wanted to share! It's astonishing how much we can learn about our bodies by checking out our poo. It's also crazy how many of us are constipated or have an unhealthy gut, but we don't know because nobody dares to talk about it.

Be brave, look behind you, and check it out!

Observe the colour, shape, texture and odour of your stools. Notice what is normal for you; any sudden changes can indicate a negative or positive effect of food and lifestyle choices.

Texture and odour

For me, these are the most important indicators of health. In Ayurveda, poo should not have a strong smell. It should be unnoticeable. If your stools are foul-smelling, your digestive organs (liver, supporting organs and GI tract) are toxically overloaded. Something in your diet or lifestyle, or both, needs to be addressed.

Texture: stools should have the consistency of toothpaste. When they are sticky, and dirty the walls of the toilet bowl, this is a sign of toxic overload. Ancient medics believed that our stools should come out cleanly (so there shouldn't be much when we wipe). They should be smooth and flow softly. Their texture should be soft enough to travel through us without pain, yet hard enough to maintain their shape when expelled.

Odour: when stools are foul-smelling and look greasy or frothy, this is usually a sign of congested liver, toxic overload and improper digestion. Check out the TOTE tips (p.168–9) to start lifting the weight off your liver, gallbladder and pancreas. Every chapter in this book will help to protect and encourage healthy liver and bowel functioning!

Shape: the shape of our stool should be robust and healthy-looking – like a banana, not a pencil. Our intestines are flexible and much larger than we think. If our stools are thin and long, it's a good idea to start packing in high-fibre foods to increase the bulk of our stool. Fibre is so important because it cleanses the intestinal lining as it passes through. Some people have thick plaque lining their inner intestinal wall – the more soluble fibre we consume the bulkier our stools are and the better job we do of eliminating waste from our gut!

Pebble-shaped stools means you are lacking fibre in your diet and can also be a sign of constipation.

Mucus

If you have noticeable mucus, a jelly-like substance, in your stools this could be a sign of inflammation. Alkalizing your diet and cutting the crap is a good start.

Colour

In general, our stools should be a shade of brown (not yellow). If your stool turns green, which mine sometimes do, this is usually because you're doing a great job of eating lots of leafy green veggies like rocket, kale and your green juice. Thumbs up if that's the case!

POO IS GREAT FEEDBACK

Generally, stools should be expelled with little effort or discomfort. When you're detoxing, it's natural to have detox symptoms, like diarrhoea or foul-smelling stools. But on a long-term basis, use your stools as a way of keeping yourself in check. It's a great way for you to understand what's happening inside! Of course, always see a doctor if you suspect something is wrong.

THE LITTLE AND BIG TOILET

There are many different euphemisms for pooing, from "going to the loo" to "number two". My favourite is "a visit to the big toilet". When we stop going to the big toilet and evacuating our bowels it means:

* *Water is reabsorbed, making stools hard and more difficult to eliminate.*
* *As our stools harden they damage the lining of our large intestines due to stagnation.*
* *Carbohydrate and sugar fermentation causes stinky gases.*
* *Animal-derived foods can putrefy in our gut.*
* *Fats become rancid, which allows toxins to be reabsorbed into the body, causing gas, constipation, headaches, heartburn and other serious conditions.*

As stools get stuck in the intestines over weeks and sometimes even years, water is reabsorbed and they harden, forming a plaque lining. This can lead to us no longer absorbing nutrients, as our digested food can't access the intestinal lining. This also causes our intestinal walls to harden as they lack nutrition, life and movement.

An impacted colon that doesn't evacuate enough can be carrying 5kg of faecal matter! Instead of the intestines absorbing nutrients from our food, toxins are absorbed from our waste.

We don't really talk about pooing. And because of that, most people with elimination issues don't even know it. A good friend of mine is a top expert and doctor for royal families and several celebrities worldwide. Only the other day, when he was on holiday with his thirteen-year-old son, he noticed his son wasn't going to the "big toilet" regularly. Little did he know, his own son was going only twice a week! Even some health experts don't talk about this at home with their children. We need to start talking about our "big toilet" visits.

Our digestive system is like that of a herbivore. It's not designed to deal with large amounts of meat. Meat can putrefy in our colon as it spends too long inside the wiggly paths of our large intestine. Eat less of it and you might feel better.

CONSTIPATION

Going to the loo at least once a day is essential.

Let's face it. Constipation is a growing problem. Because our intestines are so central to our immunity, if they are clogged, this will likely be detrimental to our vitality and joy, creating emotional, physical and mental stagnation and stress. If you're going less than once a day, please try any of the six tips above until you have your bowels moving regularly once a day! I can't emphasis enough how important this is. I used to notice that symptoms of flu or sickness only appeared when I had not been to the toilet for two days. The minute I realized this, I began making my big toilet visits a major priority for my wellbeing. Since then my vitality has drastically improved.

All the tips in this chapter encourage daily detoxification on every level, including going to the big toilet. In fact, every principle in this book, the foundations of MorLife Wellness, supports a healthy gut and thus a strong immune system.

JUICING 101

Green juice = instant medicine that takes little effort to digest/absorb. Green smoothie = fibre-filled, with a broom effect that cleans your gut.

Drinking your vegetables will literally change your life! Green juices are the most consistent part of my daily routine. If you do nothing else, drink your breakfast. I like to stick to pure vegetables, with tasty veggies like cucumbers and celery, which make a perfect base.

Because juice has no fibre, the body can quickly absorb the vitamins, minerals, proteins and enzymes directly into the bloodstream – it's instantaneous nutrition, alkalinity and oxygen for our cells. Juice from vegetable cells is in the perfect form for the cells of our body to absorb it. When we drink water, our bodies need to prepare it for cellular absorption; when we drink vegetable juice, it is already prepared and therefore is easily absorbed. Drink your juice immediately once you've made it to get maximum nutrients.

JUICING FRUITS

Due to the high sugar content in fruit, I prefer to eat it rather than drink it, because the fibre helps to slow down sugar absorption.

Juicing Tips

At first, make your juice your way; it has to be tasty enough so that you DRINK IT! Whatever you drink is good. Once it's a habit, slowly wean yourself off the sugary fruits until it contains more veggies than fruit.

Leafy green juice options

Other optional greens I love are kale, parsley, coriander, watercress, rocket and dandelion. Be adventurous and add any of these to your green juice or smoothie to increase their nutrient content. If you keep the ingredients in the fridge, it will be fresh and chilled when made.

Six tips for keeping healthy bowel movements and preventing a bunch of diseases:

1. Fluids: Purified water, green juices and smoothies! Keeping your gut well hydrated ensures it will keep things moving smoothly and surely right out of you!

2. Exercise: Regular exercise stimulates the digestive system and the natural contractions of our intestines (peristalsis), which creates regular elimination. It also prevents our abdominal muscles from sagging and becoming weak.

3. Good bacteria: Healthy flora (probiotics) in our gut makes up 70 per cent of our immune system. Our overall immunity is based on a battle between the good bacteria and bad bacteria in our intestines. If we keep the good guys strong and happy, we are boosting our immunity and preventing sickness.

Sources of good bacteria (probiotics):
* *fermented foods*
* *a high-quality probiotic supplement*

Keep your good bacteria happy and strong with:
* *plenty of water*
* *soluble fibre (prebiotics, which feed the probiotics)*
* *green juices and smoothies encourage the vitality of your gut flora*

4. Respond: Go to the toilet when nature calls. Suppressing this need can cause chronic constipation and many other complications. Our body is trying to create a routine, so let's respect it. Many experts suggest using a small step to lift your feet slightly when you go to the loo to emulate a squatting action. This helps to naturally eliminate the stools.

5. Fibre: Fibre is the body's superhero! It supports regular bowel movements, absorbs toxins, cholesterol and heavy metals, deactivates carcinogens, feeds the good bacteria in our gut (prebiotic action), and aids in weight loss because it fills you up and has zero calories.

|184|

However, it's important to drink sufficient fluids too. As fibre absorbs water, increasing our fibre intake without increasing fluid intake can actually cause dehydration and constipation. So, drink water and eat fibre! Here are some good sources:

SOLUBLE FIBRE	INSOLUBLE FIBRE
Sources:	Sources:
Oats	Whole grains
Apples	Nuts
Pears	Seeds
Berries	Dark leafy greens
Flaxseeds	Celery
Beans	Cabbage
Peas	Broccoli
Lentils	Root vegetable skins
	Onions
Action in the body:	Dried fruit
Absorbs water	Action in the body:
Forms a gel in your intestines, which creates smoother transit	Does not absorb water
When it absorbs water, it increases in size and softly attaches to impurities on the gut walls.	Acts as a broom though your intestines
Helps to reduce cholesterol.	Helps keep you regular

6. **Relax:** Finding time to relax is so important to the functioning of our bowels. If we are always "on the go", it's natural that our body will feel the stress. If we are tense, our intestinal muscles will also be tense. Exercise helps to de-stress, however it's important to engage in relaxing movement, such as yoga, if we feel like tension is present in our body.

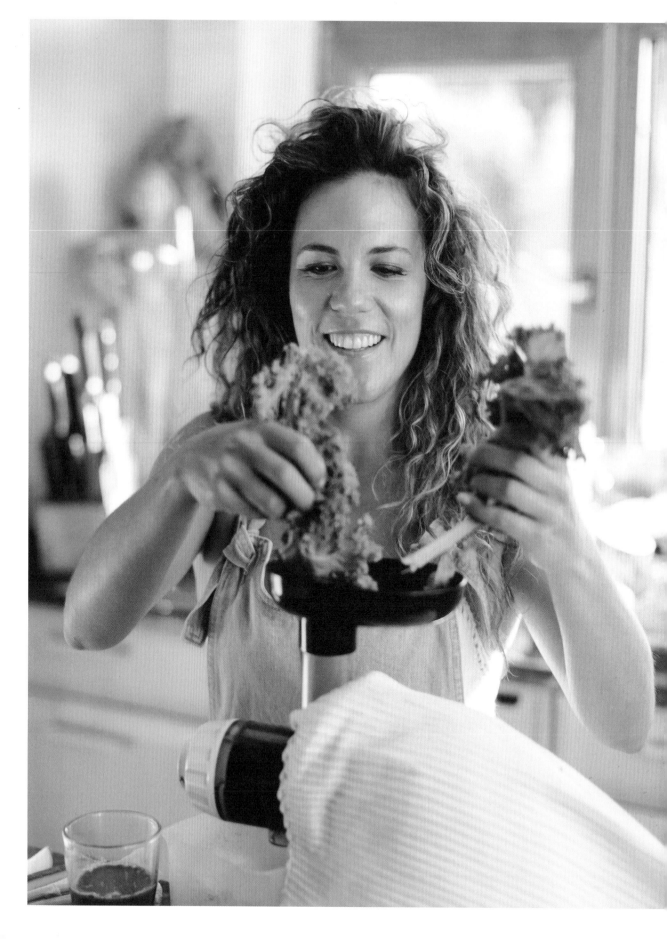

DANAH'S GREEN JUICE

Add any of the leafy greens from the leafy green list (p.73) you like to this juice. Go easy because juiced greens can be strong in flavour! Add mint and ginger for more taste.

Ingredients

* 2–3 celery stalks
* 1 large cucumber (peel if not organic)
* a handful of spinach or kale
* a handful of sprouts of your choice
* a small handful of parsley
* juice of ½ a lemon (add at the end for flavour)
* for beginners or children: ½–1 green apple (peel if not organic)

Juice all the ingredients in a juicer. A slow masticating juicer gives the best quality juice.

Drink immediately after juicing.

MEAN GREEN SMOOTHIE

Remember to chew this smoothie. It's filled with fibre. Chewing helps stimulate digestive enzyme production and will aid its digestion and the absorption of its nutrients.

Ingredients

* 1–2 cups of water
* a big handful of spinach
* a big handful of lettuce
* 1 apple, chopped
* 1 pear, chopped
* 2–3 celery stalks, chopped
* 1 banana (can be frozen)
* juice of ½ lemon

Pour the water into a blender and add the spinach and lettuce. Blend until smooth. Add the apple, pear and celery. Blend until smooth. Finally, add the banana and lemon juice, blend once more and enjoy straight away.

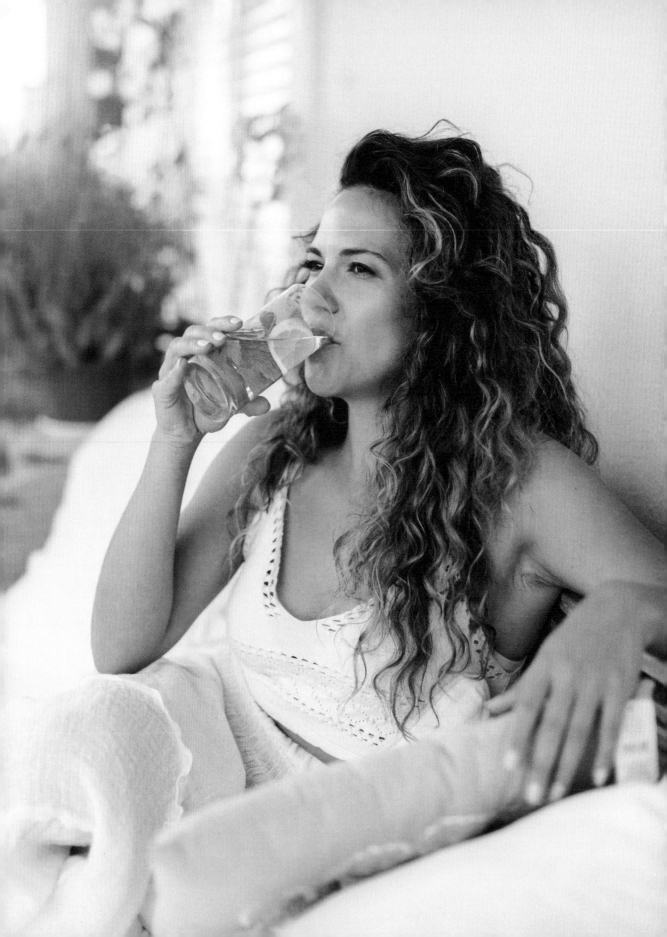

> *"Water is the driving force of all nature."*
>
> Leonardo da Vinci

Chapter 10

DRINK REAL WATER

THE TRUE VALUE OF WATER

WATER IS UNDERRATED. SO MANY OF US TAKE IT FOR GRANTED. WATER IS SECOND ONLY TO AIR IN ORDER OF IMPORTANCE FOR LIFE. WE CAN LIVE FOR THIRTY DAYS WITHOUT EATING, BUT WE CANNOT LIVE SEVENTY-TWO HOURS WITHOUT WATER. OUR BODY IS MADE UP OF 70–80 PER CENT WATER, AND IF WE DON'T KEEP IT THAT WAY, WE ARE SETTING OURSELVES UP FOR DISASTER.

The sad news is that we, as a world community, have contaminated our water supply.

This chapter emphasizes the importance of drinking real water. In short, it's to remind you that life will just be better if you make it a habit to drink fresh, pure water all day, every day. After we've pinned that down, we dive deeper into how we can begin to protect and recover our once-clean water.

"Pure water is the world's first and foremost medicine."
Slovakian proverb

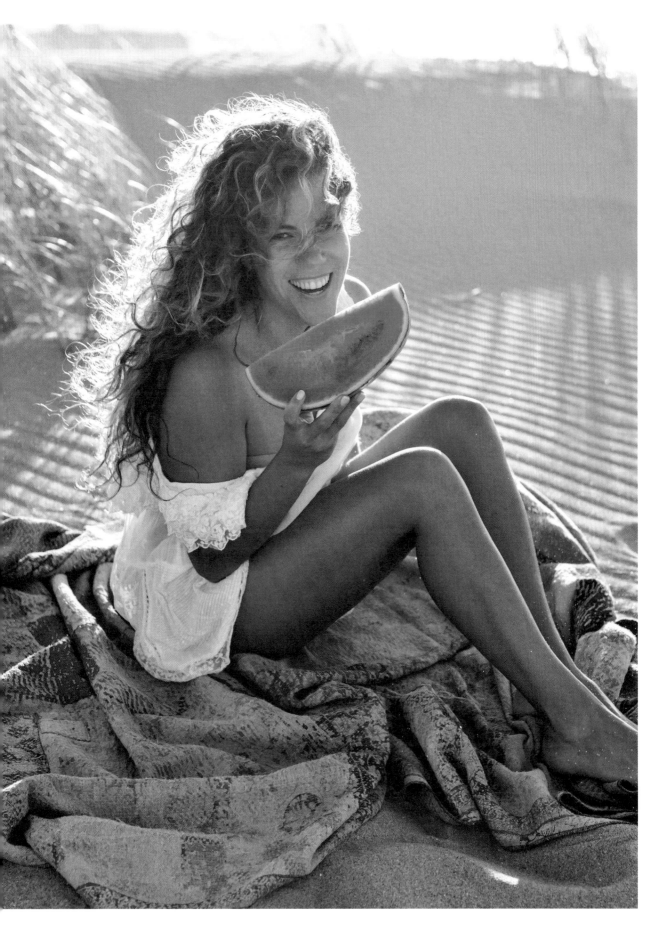

WHY DRINK WATER?

11 miraculous reasons to drink more (good-quality alkaline) water:

1. **"Hydrate instead of medicate!"** Next time you feel a sickness coming on, sip water! Microorganisms such as bacteria cannot survive in an environment flooded with alkaline water. Alkaline water can carry minerals your body needs, like calcium, magnesium and potassium. Squeeze lemon or lime juice into your water to boost its alkalinity.

|192|

2. **Increases energy, concentration and reduces fatigue.** Since your brain is 83 per cent water, drinking it helps you think and concentrate better. It increases your energy and mood, and makes you more alert.

3. **Promotes weight loss.** Water fills you up, naturally reduces hunger, raises your metabolism, improves digestion and has zero calories! (Drink it away from meals, not while you eat, as it dilutes your enzymes).

4. **Flushes out toxins**. Water helps to flush out toxins and digestive waste. It eliminates waste through sweat and urination, helping the body to TOTE, avoiding toxic build-up.

5. **Glowing smooth skin.** Water is a natural skin moisturizer. Proper hydration keeps your skin fresh, soft, smooth and glowing.

6. **Keeps you regular.** When your gut is hydrated, everything runs smoothly. Keep the H20 coming and prevent your stools from hardening, leading to constipation.

7. **Prevents and relieves headaches.** The first thing I do when my head starts to hurt is drink water. Headaches and migraines are often caused by dehydration.

8. **Reduces water retention and improves circulation.** Water retention and swelling can be due to dehydration.

9. **Prevents cramps and sprains.** Our joints are lubricated and muscles are kept elastic by water.

10. **Mood booster.** When the body is functioning at its best, you will feel vitality, strength and peace, hoo-ha!

11. **Save money. Water is FREE!** Even if you choose bottled or filtered water, it's usually cheaper than high-sugar drinks and juices.

WATER, THE FOUNTAIN OF LIFE

Water is my favourite drink, and it has been since I was a child. My parents did a great job of making sure that's all we had at home. It worked. I love water. (Okay, I love artisanal beer, too, but water is always my first choice!) Scientists have been studying water for decades and there are still aspects of it they cannot fully understand. It's a magical element essential for the planet, the environment and all forms of life. Water covers our planet, making it possible for us to live on it. This marks the difference between planet Earth and other planets. In our bodies, water is essential for almost every function. It protects our organs, transports nutrients and eliminates acidic toxic waste through our urine, bowels and sweat. It also increases oxygen in our blood and keeps our skin soft, young and supple. Research has found that failing to drink enough water can shrink your grey matter (brain), making it harder to think! *What?*

Our vital organs and tissues are basically made of water:
* *Muscles and heart: 75 per cent*
* *Brain and kidneys: 83 per cent*
* *Lungs: 86 per cent*
* *Blood: 94 per cent*
* *Eyes: 95 per cent!*

Just 90 minutes of steady sweating can shrink the brain as much as a year of ageing. Our bodies need as much water in cold weather as they do in warm weather, and just as much when we are sleeping as when we're awake. **A 5 per cent drop in body fluids will cause a 25–30 per cent loss of energy in most people.**

Properly hydrating the body with good water is the quickest and easiest way to feel stronger and more vital.

WATER AND DEHYDRATION

Headaches or dry mouth and skin are some of the most common signs of dehydration. Most of us are chronically dehydrated most of the time and don't even know it. No wonder so many of us are tired and can't think straight.

On average, people only get approximately one litre of fluid a day, most of it being from acidic coffee, tea and sugary drinks, which rob the body of water and nutrients.

Early signs of dehydration:
* *Headaches (including light headaches)*
* *Foggy thinking*
* *Short-term memory problems*
* *Difficulty focusing*
* *Cold hands and feet*

* *Anxiety*
* *Irritation*
* *Depression*
* *Sugar cravings*
* *Cramps*
* *Dark yellow urine*

Signs of severe dehydration:

* *Acid reflux heartburn*
* *Joint and back pain*
* *Migraines*
* *Fibromyalgia*
* *Constipation*
* *Colitis*
* *Angina*

If you're feeling any of the above signs, it's time to get into a serious relationship with water. Make it a ritual, do a little dance, and get down with your water!

Urine colour can indicate dehydration. Keeping an eye on your urine can also help remind you to drink more. Ideally, urine should be a transparent light yellow colour, like straw. If it's a darker amber yellow, it means you need to drink more water.

Drink even if you're not thirsty, because remember, feeling thirsty means you're already dehydrated. Sip water throughout the day, rather than chugging down a litre twice a day. Our bodies are unable to absorb large amounts of water at

once. Drinking a litre all at once can overwork your kidneys. Avoid drinking too much water during meals because it dilutes your digestive enzymes. Finally, if you're drinking out of plastic bottles, never leave them in the car or the sun because the heat causes the plastic to leach into the water.

How much water?

You should be drinking between 1.5–3 litres (2.5–5 pints) of water per day depending on your weight and size. I carry around a large 1.5 litre bottle with me every day, and I make sure it's finished at the end of the day before I get home.

Here's a formula:
Drink X litres/fl oz of pure, mildly alkaline water:
X litres = your weight kg/33.8
X fl oz = body weight (lbs.)/2
1 cup = 240ml/8 fluid ounces

The habit of drinking water is the most important thing to focus on here. Once we have pinned down the habit, we can start to look into what sort of water is best for our vitality. Since we're pretty much made up of water, we might as well be drinking the best kind.

Make drinking water part of your routine:

1. **Always drink a big glass of lemon water first thing in the morning,** before anything else. And a few hours before you go to bed.

2. **Drink your green juice.** Get half a litre of water straight from plant cells to your cells. This alkaline water can be immediately absorbed by your cells! It's a direct transfusion of live water.

3. **Have a second big glass of water** at least one hour before lunch.

4. **Keep a jug of water or a water bottle on your desk at work,** mark it with time-oriented goals, and get competitive with yourself.

5. **Invest in a good-quality BPA-free plastic or glass water bottle** and take it with you everywhere you go.

6. **Spice up you water experience.** If you find plain H2O boring, add lemon, cucumber, apple or ginger slices for flavour. Mint, lemongrass or parsley are also refreshing and great during the summer. Crush the leaves softly in your hands to release more aroma into the water. Herbal teas are also infused water, and warm water is great for your digestion and immunity, so make a large thermos and keep drinking throughout the day – I can't work without a thermos of herbal tea!

7. **Make it fun.** Choose a fun cup to drink from or a cool straw – whatever gets you drinking. My friend Daniel uses a Spiderman cup to remind him that superheroes drink their water!

8. **Take a sip whenever you pass by a drinking fountain.**

9. **Download a water drinking app and drink accordingly!**

10. **If you feel hungry, have a glass of water.** Hunger and thirst activate the same mechanism in the body, so next time you think you're hungry, you might just be thirsty.

11. **Eat your water.** Many raw vegetables and fruits are full of water and the veggies are richer in alkaline water. Juice them or eat them as snacks instead of biscuits – cucumber, celery, radishes, tomatoes, red bell peppers, watermelon, grapes and strawberries. Once they're cooked, they lose much of their water content, so have them raw.

WATER QUALITY

Our natural sources of water are becoming increasingly contaminated with pesticides, pharmaceutical chemicals, plastic residues, toxins, parasites and more. Keep calm and keep drinking water. Before we get into the details of each water source, here are a few general rules.

1. **Drink neutral to slightly alkaline water.** Check the pH and ensure it is above 7 (neutral). In an ideal world, water should be at least pH7 neutral, but most tap and even bottled water is acidic. Water in nature is slightly alkaline due to the alkaline minerals present in it. This is the best form of water. Check the pH of water with pH strips, and for bottled water, it always appears on the nutrient info label.

2. **Do not drink fluoridated water.** Fluoride is a neurotoxin that attacks our brain cells. Although it has been banned in most European countries, water fluoridation still takes place in many countries around the world. Fluoride is a recognized neurotoxin that can cause death even at very low doses. It is proven to be highly toxic for the brain. Governments add it to tap water to improve dental health, but it is known to cause more harm than good. Make sure you are not drinking fluoridated water. Ask your water supply company for their water tests. If your water is fluoridated, ensure you purify it before drinking and don't use it for baby bottles.

3. **Avoid being contaminated by getting informed about your tap water source.** Get a copy of the water-quality report from the company supplying your tap water. Find out where your tap water comes from. For example, check if your water is fluoridated or contains any local contaminants, such as pesticides and heavy metals. Check out the list of contaminants to avoid on the next page.

4. **Vary your water source.** All water sources have minor contaminants; by varying them, we lower our risk of accumulation.

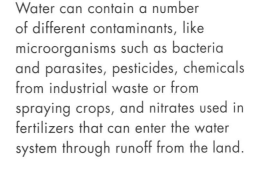

Water can contain a number of different contaminants, like microorganisms such as bacteria and parasites, pesticides, chemicals from industrial waste or from spraying crops, and nitrates used in fertilizers that can enter the water system through runoff from the land.

Once, spring water and wells were our only water sources, but nowadays there are so many ways to drink water, from tap water and filters to bottled water and sophisticated purification systems. It can be confusing to know what's real and good.

|197|

WHAT TO AVOID IN YOUR WATER

The main things we want to filter out are:

1. Chlorine and disinfecting byproducts (more dangerous to health than chlorine)

2. Toxins and acids

3. Pharmaceutical chemicals

4. Heavy metals – e.g. lead from old pipes

5. Pesticides

6. Local contaminants (see your local water report)

WHAT KIND OF WATER IS BEST TO DRINK?

TAP WATER

The positives of tap water are that it's free and sustainable. However, the quality of your tap water depends on the country, municipality and area it's supplied from. Most tap water is disinfected and purified with chlorine and chemicals, which have been linked with serious health complications. It can also contain bacteria, parasites, and pharmaceutical chemicals, pesticides and heavy metals, including lead and copper from pipes. Avoid lead contamination by only using cold water for consumption and let the tap run a bit before using the water (ideally, if you know your building has old lead piping, you should insist they be replaced with non-toxic new materials). Other contaminants in our water supply might include arsenic, aluminum (closely linked to Alzheimer's), prescription, over-the-counter and recreational drugs, fluoride, and disinfectant byproducts.

WATER FILTERS

Water distiller: Distilled water is boiled and evaporated, losing both its minerals and impurities in the process. Because it no longer contains its naturally alkaline minerals, the water becomes acidic. This can mean it then draws minerals right out of our body, leaving us more acidic. It's a good way to get pure water, but being mineral-less means it can have adverse effects if you drink too much of it long term.

Reverse osmosis filter: These filters force water through membranes that remove larger particles, including pollutants and minerals. This is commonly used to protect pipes from calcification residues. But again, these remove alkalizing minerals which can leave the water acidic.

FILTERED TAP WATER

I like the idea of filtering tap water because it provides inexpensive purified water that is also environmentally friendly!

Filters efficiently remove more water contaminants than many other techniques, including chlorine and other dangerous disinfecting byproducts (DPAs) present in tap water. Water filters also leave natural minerals in the water that both distillation and reverse osmosis methods remove. There are several types of tap water filtration systems available on the market. Some filters are more efficient at removing contaminants than others. Research and find out how the filtration system functions, ensuring that it filters harmful contaminants present in your local tap water rather than the alkaline minerals. Make sure you check them out properly before being seduced into expensive hardware!

BOTTLED WATER

I've drunk a lot of bottled water. It definitely helps me keep hydrated on the go, wherever I travel to. Nowadays, we can find great hard plastic or glass travel bottles

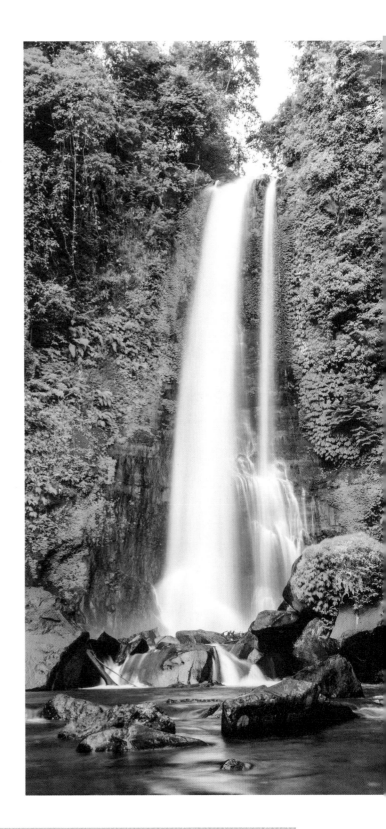

that keep water safe from plastic contamination. Bottled water is not necessarily more pure than purified tap water, as there are no specific regulatory bodies checking their quality, although we can control mineral content and pH of bottled water. So, if you are travelling or on the go, always choose mineral or spring water with a pH of 7 or higher. Choose local bottled water and reuse the bottles. If you reuse the bottle to drink water, make sure you clean it well. Research says that it's bacteria and fungi that are actually more dangerous to us than the plastic leaching in. So when reusing water bottles it's important to wash them well and let them dry between uses.

Cleaning your reusable water bottle

Whether it's metallic, hard plastic or glass, when we are drinking out of a reusable water bottle it's so important to clean it properly on a daily basis. Use bicarbonate soda or vinegar and soak your water bottles overnight. If it's metallic you can boil the bottle to sterilize it. I have a glass bottle at my desk which I use only as a pitcher to pour the water into a glass. This means I only have to wash the glass daily – it's easier!

SPRING WATER

My favourite! Spring water is nature's perfect form of living water. It's the earth's gift to us. Spring water comes from aquifers and underground lakes deep under the ground. This water has been underground for hundreds, sometimes thousands, of years. Spring water is pure and naturally mineralized, making it slightly alkaline. Unlike tap water and bottled water, spring water is not industrially processed. It's real! In an ideal world, it is the best water to consume. Findaspring.com can help you locate springs near you and keep you quenched with nature's best water source. However, since we're so good at messing with nature's perfect balance, our non-biodegradable pesticides, chemicals, toxins and more can leach into our underground water reservoirs, so before jumping to drink from a spring water source, find out if there are any harmful contaminants in that spring.

Drinking slightly alkaline water will help to neutralize acidity in the body and can reduce the amount of free radical damage. It will also help to keep your bones and teeth strong. We can make our water slightly more alkaline by adding lemon juice to it or a tablespoon of organic apple cider vinegar.

PROTECT OUR NATURAL WATER SUPPLIES

How many of us know where our running tap water comes from? Most of the world depends on clean water from lakes and rivers, but most of these lakes and rivers are being seriously polluted and depleted to the extent that we may be facing water shortage within the next 10 years. Many experts believe the next world war could be over clean drinking water.

We can't afford to destroy our drinking water sources, but we're doing so unknowingly. We've heard about saving water – taking shorter showers, for example – but there are many more things we can do to stop polluting, contaminating and depleting our natural groundwater supplies that take no extra effort.

Just because it disappears, doesn't mean it goes away.

Seven ways to reduce water pollution and conserve and protect our local ground water supply:

1. **Think twice about disposing detergents and medications down the sink.** What we throw down our sink or toilet will eventually land in our lakes, rivers and tap water.

2. **Choose natural, phosphate-free soaps and detergents** that are biodegradable. And avoid the use of bleach.

3. **Avoid the use of pesticides, herbicides and fertilizers** (ideally, choose organic foods and refrain from using these in your garden). These substances don't decompose in nature – they continue to work their "death sentences" into our rivers, lakes and natural water reserves.

4. **Throw away all oils safely.** Put them in specific oil recycling bins and not down the drain.

5. **Reduce your consumption of animal foods.** Forests, grasslands and wetlands are nature's water filters. Deforestation occurs to create feeding ground for cattle, and more than 70 per cent of water withdrawn from nature goes to agriculture.

6. **Turn off the tap while brushing your teeth.**

7. **Always run full loads of dishes and laundry.**

|201|

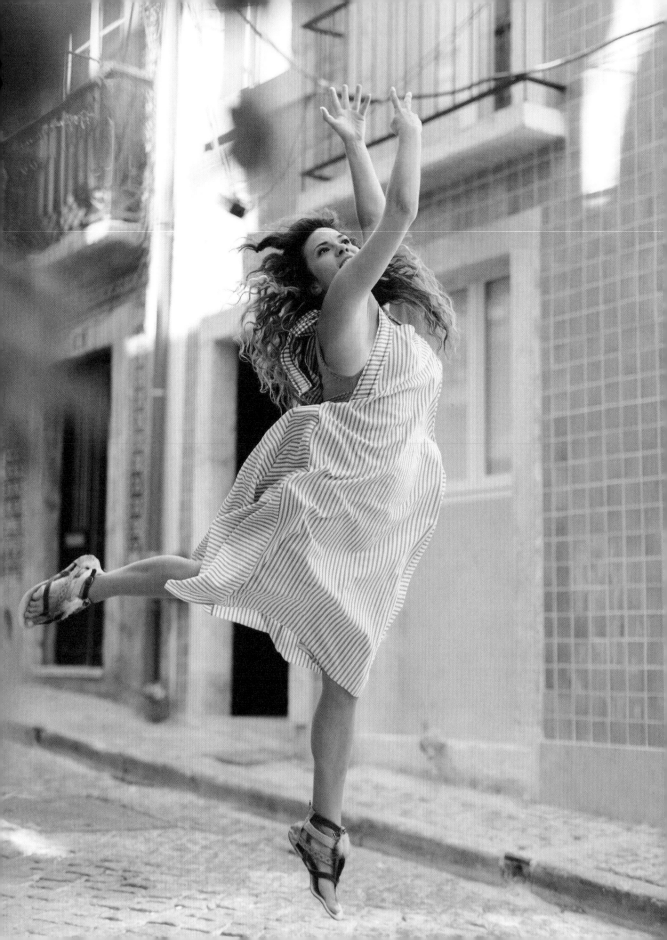

Move, and you might move out of your own way.

Chapter 11

DANCE.
EVERY DAY

LET'S GET MOVING!

THE DESIGN OF OUR BODY IS CREATED FOR MOVEMENT – EASY, NATURAL MOVEMENT. THINK ABOUT HOW ONLY ABOUT A HUNDRED YEARS AGO, MOVEMENT WAS A NORMAL PART OF OUR DAY.

We did aerobic activity by walking for transportation, we weight-lifted by working machines, toiling on the farm, taking the stairs. We were moving all the time. Today, we're pretty disconnected from this natural way of being. We drive cars, sit at desks and watch TV.

We're the first generation to hardly move. Children spend more than seven and a half hours a day in front of a screen. In fact, moving has become so far from what we consider normal, it's almost an inconvenience to move.

"I was almost anti-exercise when I began eating properly. Eating right made good sense because I lost a lot of weight. But exercise was a big stretch for me. The fact is that I struggled with exercise. I went to a gym and I started, and I can assure you that two months into it, I looked back and wondered how I ever lived without movement."

Brian Clement, PhD, author of Life Force

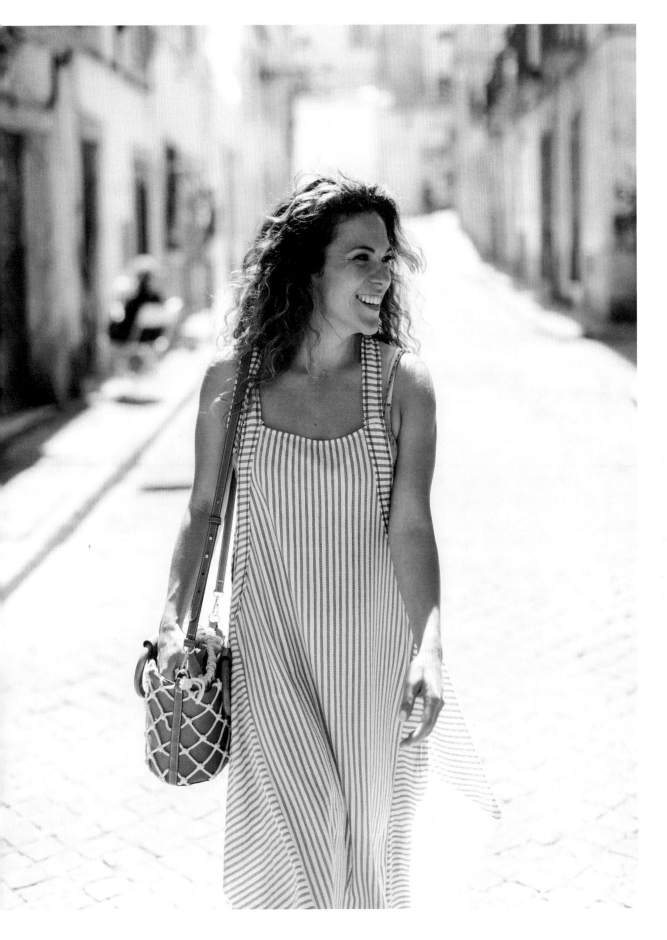

OUR BODY IS DESIGNED TO BE MOVING

Our body craves movement and is most happy when our muscles are used, stretched, joints are lubricated, organs are massaged, and the lymph system is pumped by our muscle contractions.

Dr Kenneth Cooper, MD/MPH, trained the 1970 Brazilian soccer team to a World Cup victory. He scientifically proved the huge impact regular movement has on the body, stating that 35 minutes, five days a week of movement is the minimum needed for health benefits.

"As a pro dancer, when I go on holiday, I feel like something is missing. I have to find ways to be active. Dancing is my healthy addiction."

Vanda Gameiro, professional dancer

Exercise creates positive vibrations, makes us feel alive, creates happy chemicals and gives us a high.
When we exercise, our body releases feel-good chemicals into our brain. These are responsible for that "high" that follows a workout. These chemicals are powerful mind- and mood-boosting substances: **dopamine** – the pleasure chemical often associated with orgasms; **endorphins** – which create euphoric feelings in the body, decrease stress, decrease appetite, improve immune response, and block pain receptors in our brain; and **serotonin** – a natural mood booster and the chemical responsible for happiness and restful sleep.

Our personality changes when we have a body we feel good in. Sometimes a lack of exercise creates stagnation in the body and mind. Physical movement is the best way to get ourselves unstuck. If you're stuck in your mind, moving will get you out of the mind and into your body. If you're stuck in your body, moving will get energy flowing and unblock tension.

BENEFITS OF REGULAR MOVEMENT

PHYSICAL BENEFITS

1. Eliminates heaviness and stiffness in the body, creates flexibility, lightness, smoothness and flow
2. Increases circulation in all parts of the body, improving cell nutrition, oxygenation and detoxification
3. Increases toxic elimination and prevents toxic build-up in organs
4. Pumps the lymph system, the biggest filtering system in the body
5. Causes sweating, which cleanses skin pores and improves microcirculation to face skin and eyes
6. Improves organ, respiratory and immunological function
7. Reduces and prevents infections and inflammatory conditions
8. Stimulates the immune system by increasing response capacity of immune cells. Regulates and balances weight
9. Balances and improves sexual vitality
10. Reduces risk of major diseases; prevents heart attacks
11. Improves energy, mood, sleep, digestion
12. Prevents cellulite
13. Relieves stress
14. Balances hormone levels (regular aerobic exercise)
15. Improves heart and lung function
16. Rejuvenates: keeps us young
17. Relieves hot flashes
18. Protects men's health (pelvic exercises help prevent erectile dysfunction and possibly benign prostate enlargement)
19. Stimulates the growth of new brain cells
20. Improves brain function
21. Dance specifically has been shown to prevent dementia and Parkinson's

EMOTIONAL & PSYCHOLOGICAL BENEFITS

1. Boosts self-esteem
2. Reduces stress
3. Reduces anxiety and feelings of depression
4. Improves memory and mental functioning
5. Reduces incidence of depression; it has helped relieve depression as effectively as antidepressant medication (for many)
6. Improves mood
7. Releases emotional tension
8. Increases cognitive capacity and memory
9. Creates serotonin, the happy chemical often used in antidepressants
10. Improves sleep
11. Clarity of thought, desire, and vigor; reduces anxiety, stress and depression

What if I'm not a gym person?

I'm not a gym person. However, finally, after many years of time-consuming experimentation, I have finally found my favourite form of movement. Now I've got a few tips to help you find yours.

Physical movement/activity has to be fun and enjoyable. Otherwise, you're less likely to stick to it and make it a habit.

Think about what you loved to do as a kid. Dance, bike, run, hike? Be creative and revisit some of those fun activities you used to love.

"Fitness is a journey, not a destination; you must continue for the rest of your life."
Dr. Kenneth Cooper

My story

I was a very active kid growing up. My sport was competitive league basketball, but I got injured and had to stop. I got depressed and started coaching basketball, but I wasn't moving. I put on weight and started to feel sad and frustrated. I sprang from sport to pool to gym, trying to find some form of movement that would bring some life back into me. It took me three years of experimenting to find movement I loved, and then another year to make a regular habit of it.

We all love to move. Look at kids – climbing trees, jumping and running around. It's in our nature. **The pressure of the gym, being fit, or fitting in, are annoying and unhelpful,** so let's throw them out and change our perspective on movement. Let's try and see movement as something our body craves and loves. Our body is like a rusty bicycle that needs to be used, to be lubricated. Our body is also very forgiving, and even if it has been years since we properly moved, once we start again, it does everything to get strong and stronger, slowly but surely.

My passion for physical activity has finally landed me home. Dancing is my form of self-expression, my medicine! You can dance anywhere and everywhere. Put some music on every day and dance till you break a sweat! Dance not only gets you moving, it also gets you to express yourself from the inside out in a wonderful way. And between us, you don't have to know how to dance, you just have to move to a beat.

E-MOTION AND DANCE

When we move, and especially when we truly give into the music and allow it to express itself through our movement – this is real dance – we are forced out of our own head and into our body. Not only does our body accumulate tension and trauma but this tension can remain in the body for life. We're talking about emotional traumas and tensions that turn into physical (psychosomatic) lesions. Moving your body freely through dance can help to release stuck emotions, moving them out of your body, creating space and a lot of relief!

DANCING AND THE BRAIN

Dancing increases cognitive acuity at all ages.

A study that researched the beneficial effects of different activities – from walking, swimming, dancing and jogging to playing cards, cross-word puzzles or reading – found that only dancing offered any protection against dementia, Alzheimer's and other brain-related conditions.

The greatest risk reduction of any activity studied, cognitive or physical, was dance at 76 per cent! A 2003 study in the *New England Journal of Medicine* by researchers at the Albert Einstein College of Medicine discovered that dance can decidedly improve brain health. Dancing involves both a mental effort and social interaction, and this type of stimulation helps reduce the risk of dementia.

Dancing develops new neural connections and pathways – making us more intelligent!

Dance requires us to connect our mind and our body – something that is increasingly rare nowadays. We are either at a desk, using just our mind, or at the gym with headphones on, working our bodies disconnectedly. There are few activities that connect so many areas of the brain at the same moment.

JUST DANCE

Physical movement was part of a normal day back when we lived more in tune with nature. Don't allow the development of technology to build a bigger gap between you and your body's basic needs! Find an activity that gets your body moving and schedule it into your week.

If you find it hard to schedule in time for physical movement, next time you organize a coffee appointment with a friend, go for a walk together! Or park your car further away from your destination to give you a bit of a walk. Always choose the path that gets you moving.

YOU CAN PUSH YOUR MIND, BUT DON'T PUSH YOUR BODY

Listen to your body when you move. My best lessons have come from listening to my body.

For seven years, I trained basketball six times a week and never had a body I was happy with. I felt uncomfortable and didn't like looking in the mirror. I got injured (numerous times), was forced to stop playing and put on weight. One day, I got tricked into a Pilates class, and within one week, my body had changed shape – without pain or any sweaty exercise. I was shocked, yet impressed – how was this possible? No pain? By recruiting core muscles for proper posture, I was changing my silhouette. I couldn't believe it!

"No pain, no gain" is outdated. Exercise should not hurt. It should feel natural, even if we have to force ourselves to move, we should always respect our physical limits. We don't need to push ourselves to get results. We can build our strength gradually by walking, swimming, even gardening and cleaning the house. Many of us push ourselves past our limits and are then forced to stop through injury or breakdown. Make the journey pleasurable and steady by tuning into your body and respecting its limits.

TOO MUCH OR TOO LITTLE

Respect your limits. **You can push your mind, but don't push your body.** In Ayurveda, exercising beyond our capacity can do more harm than good. Every time I try to push myself to exercise harder or pull more weight, I put on weight. I get tense and become bloated. Psychologically, it is essential to enjoy the movement you do. If you feel depressed, put on some music and dance! Sometimes we do need to force ourselves to go for a walk or get to a gym class, but always take small steps so that you are taking your body with you.

NOT ALL EXERCISE IS ONE SIZE FITS ALL

Listen to your body. If you feel heavy, lethargic and depressed, aerobic exercise, like a run or swim, could be a good idea. If you feel anxious, nervous and worried, try a stretching, yoga or Pilates class that's grounding and calming. Find movement that balances your mind and body at the same time. Stretching releases tension in our muscles and calms the mind. It is alkalizing!

Everyone benefits from mild aerobic alkaline physical activity.

Only 35 minutes a day, five times a week is enough to benefit your body and mind.

Aerobic means "with oxygen". Aerobic exercise increases our body's use and flow of oxygen. When we move our body enough to break a sweat and increase our breathing, our muscles pump our lymphatic system, which speeds up toxin and acid waste elimination through our skin and breath. This alkalizes our body. This kind of alkalizing exercise is light-to-moderate intensity, such as jogging, hiking, cycling, swimming, yoga and dancing.

We know we're doing aerobic exercise when our breathing gets a bit heavier than normal, but we're not out of breath (for example, we can have a conversation while exercising, but can't easily sing a song), and when our body feels warmer as we move, but not overheated.

Anaerobic, or "without oxygen", is the opposite of aerobic. Anaerobic exercise causes the body to experience an oxygen debt which produces lactic acid. Anaerobic exercise also shuts down the lymphatic system. Many make the mistake of performing aerobic activities at too high an intensity for their current fitness level, so that it becomes anaerobic and stresses the body. Whether an exercise is alkalizing and aerobic or anaerobic and acidifying all depends on whether oxygen is available or not. If we can breathe and have a conversation, we are doing aerobic exercise!

Research confirms that people can heal their bodies from inflammatory conditions and disease eight times faster if they do consistent aerobic exercise for a minimum of 35 minutes a day, five days a week. This is incredible!

When we are making changes or implementing new, better habits into our lives, creating **the habit is more important than how you move.**

> "The habit of going to the gym is more important than what you do there. Take a magazine, go to the sauna, just go to the gym."
>
> *Terry Crews, former American NFL player and actor*

If we are creatures of habit, then perhaps just going to the gym or dance class for a social encounter might be the answer. Doing any form of physical activity in our busy day takes preparation and planning. Having to take an extra change of clothes or shoes into work can be the reason we're not active. Creating and dedicating yourself to a routine that fits your busy life is a good place to start.

13 ways to make physical movement part of your routine:

1. **Focus on the habit, not the result. You don't have to go fast, you just have to go. Let go of feelings and thoughts associated with expectations and results.**

2. **Forget the "all or nothing" attitude.** Keep it simple. You don't have to spend hours exercising. For health, it's better to move for 35 minutes a day, almost every day of the week, than less days for more time.

3. **Make goals you can achieve.** If you're unlikely to do 35 minutes, five times a week, make your own objectives that you can achieve. It's more motivating to achieve our small goals – this builds momentum! Having said that, my sister tells herself she has to go to the gym every day. That way, if she has to miss a day or two, she's still gone five times in the week. Find out what works best for you.

4. **Don't judge yourself.** Judging your body or fitness level is demotivating. Be proud that you are making small but steady steps. The fact that you care is pretty cool – decide that you are awesome!

5. **Choose movement that you enjoy.** If your physical activity is unpleasant and stressful, chances are you won't go back. Choose activities that fit your taste and lifestyle. You don't need to go to the gym because that's what most people do.

6. **Be patient.** The secret here is persistence, not strength. Don't try and force yourself to become a perfect athlete overnight. Start slowly and keep at it. Life is a long time and movement needs to be part of it forever, so it's important it feels good and not stressful.

7. **Book a PT.** Support and encouragement are always helpful. If you feel you're not doing it on your own, book a personal training session once or twice a week to help you create a habit. I did that for my dad and it worked!

8. **Schedule it.** Add your physical activity to your calendar. Make it as important as a date or a meeting.

9. **Prepare your gear the night before.** I like to keep my gym/dance bag in the car, with extra clean clothes and a swimsuit. That way, I'm always prepared. Prepare your gear the night before so that it's not a hassle in the morning.

10. **Think outside the gym.** If you find the gym inconvenient, expensive, intimidating or boring, there's a world of motion outside it! Here are just a few ideas:
    Dancing – yeah! / Hiking / Rollerblading / Yoga (active yoga)
    Paddle boarding / Horseback riding / Kayaking / Outdoor group
    jogging / Gymnastics / Martial arts / Rock climbing / Zumba
    Adult football league / Adult water polo / Fencing

11. **Make it a social event with friends or family.** Creating a ritual or habit to move with people you like is motivating as it's always fun to catch up with people that matter to you. Other people can also hold you accountable, so you're less likely to flake out.

12. **Combine your workout with a treat.** Watch your favourite TV show while you're on the treadmill or bike. Listen to an audio book as you jog or walk. Make your movement sessions a fun part of your life.

13. **The fact that you care is pretty cool** – decide that you are awesome!

BE AN ACTIVE PERSON

We don't need to solely dedicate ourselves to a single sports activity to feel active. Keeping active throughout the day is a longevity and wellness secret. Even if we spend most of our day at work or home, there are simple ways to keep up our movement levels. Think of physical activity as a lifestyle rather than a task on the weekly agenda. Here are six easy ways to sneak movement into your day to make you an active person.

1. **Find ways to add extra steps.** *Take the stairs rather than the lift or escalator. Park further away from the entrance instead of right in front. Get off the train or bus a stop earlier and walk the rest of the way. These extra steps add up.*

2. **Do the household chores and gardening**. *These chores are good workouts, especially when done at a fast pace. Sweep, dust, scrub, vacuum and hang the clothes out to dry!*

3. **Take the dog out.** *Make a habit of walking the dog or go for a stroll before or after dinner. Animals are great incentives to exercise. If you don't have a dog, animal shelters always need volunteers to exercise and socialize their dogs.*

4. **Bike or walk whenever possible,** *instead of taking the car. It's also better for the environment and helps you save on petrol.*

5. **Keep moving at work.** *Take a walk during your coffee and lunch break. Walk around to talk to co-workers instead of calling them. If you can, get a small trampoline at the office and take a movement break rather than a coffee one. Spend three minutes bouncing on the trampoline or run up and down the stairs. This will increase circulation, especially to the brain, which boosts productivity.*

6. **Move during TV adverts.** *Make watching TV more active by doing sit-ups, jumping jacks, or using arm weights during commercial breaks.*

Movement should be a pleasure not a pressure. Once I started working, my physical activities were easily bumped off my schedule if I got too busy. I'm working hard to make sure it no longer gets bumped off, because, at the end of the day, moving (not hardcore exercise) is one of the few things that really helps my body and mind stay in balance. Whatever you do, keep moving!

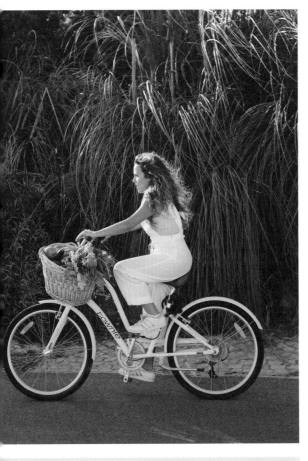
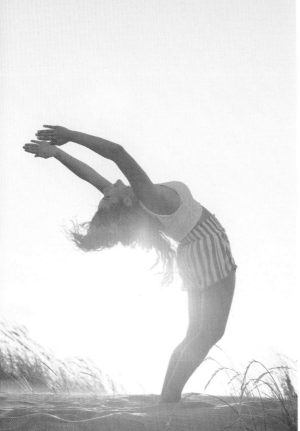
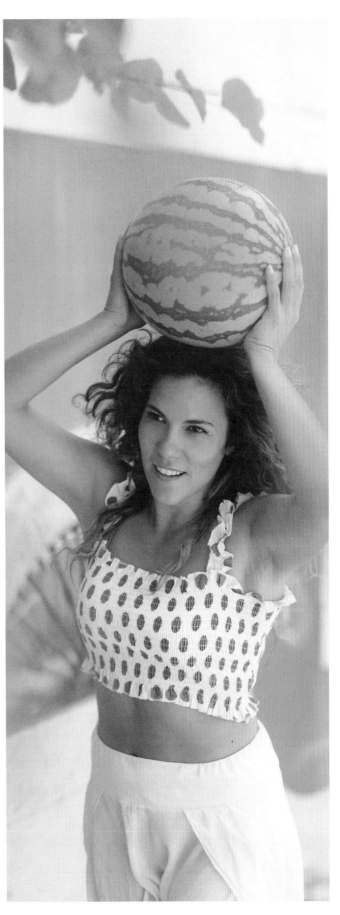

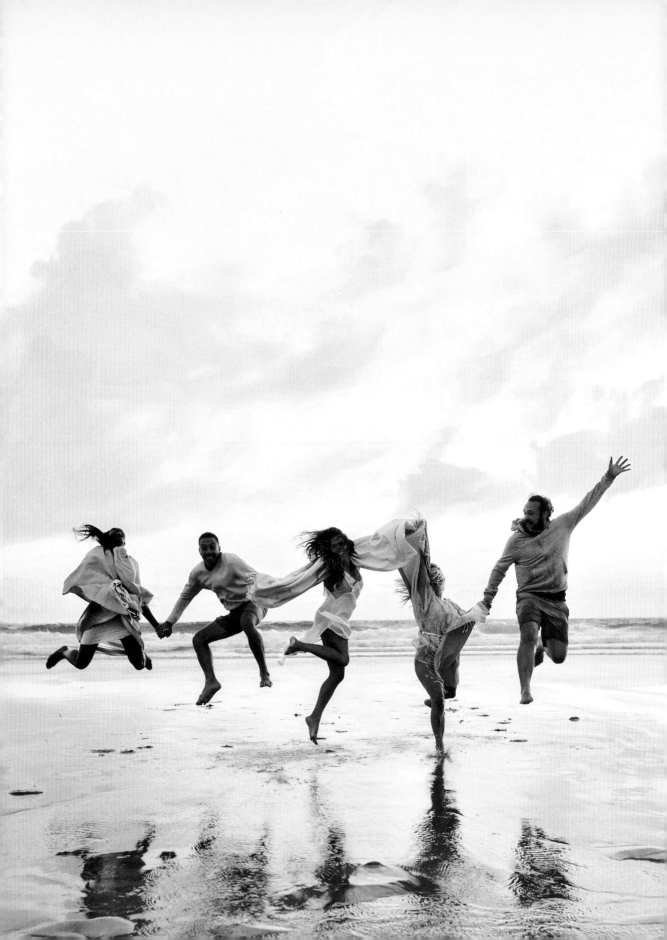

> *I was obsessed with being healthy, but I was unhappy. Something was wrong.*

Chapter 12

IT'S NOT ALL ABOUT FOOD

FEED YOUR SOUL

VITALITY AND WELLNESS ARE NOT SOLELY DEPENDENT ON WHAT GOES INTO YOUR MOUTH. YOUR RELATIONSHIPS, CAREER CHOICES, EXERCISE HABITS, AND YOUR RELATIONSHIP WITH YOURSELF HAVE A HUGE INFLUENCE ON YOUR LIFE CHOICES!

My journey in natural healthcare and food medicine has been long but extremely fun – and I'm still learning every day. One of the best lessons I've had the privilege of learning is that it's not all about food.

Part of my studies included three months at a health institute where individuals reversed all forms of catastrophic "irreversible" diseases. Our food was provided and it was of the highest quality – super organic, homegrown, homemade, raw, plant-based. Before attending, I was nervous about the diet change, but within weeks of eating this way, I noticed the difference in my body and in my skin. All puffiness and bloating was gone, and my mood was light, energetic and happy. There was only one thing wrong: my mind, my thoughts and my obsession with certain foods seemed to worsen as each day went by. I couldn't stop thinking about leaving class to go and buy coconut ice cream. These thoughts haunted me, and they took me away from enjoying myself. Ultimately, eating so strictly augmented my obsession with food.

I moved back to Portugal, where things got worse. I decided I wanted to challenge myself and continue with a plant-based diet. Portugal was new to the concept of vegetarianism, let alone veganism. I stayed home to eat because going out was almost depressing. I didn't go to the gym and started saying no to social dinners.

I was obsessed with being healthy, but I wasn't happy. Something was wrong.

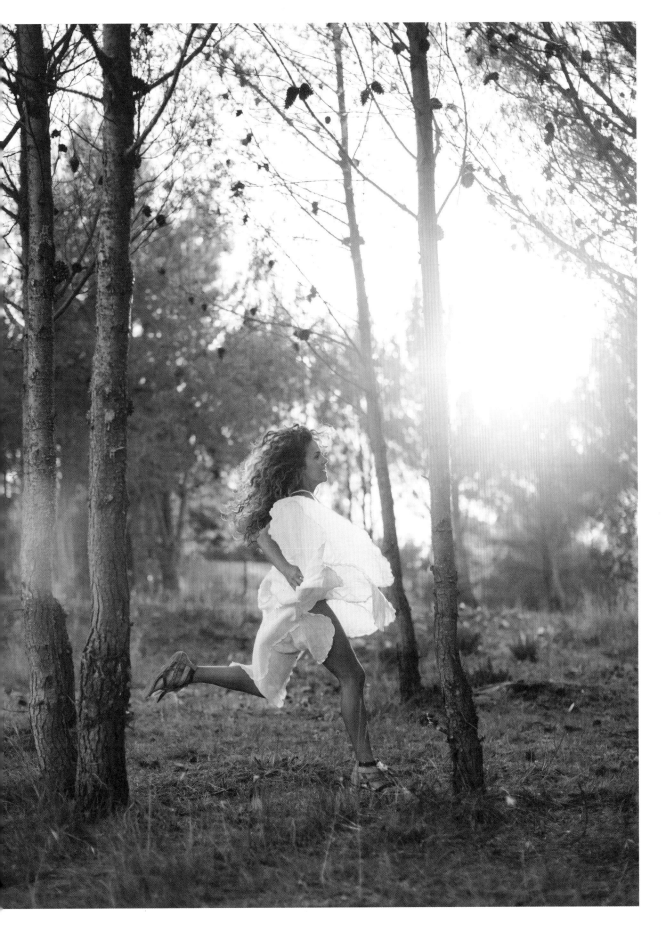

PRIMARY & SECONDARY FOODS

How do we choose what to eat? Which part of us makes these decisions?

Let me introduce you to a concept that changed my life and my perspective on nutrition. This concept is based on the idea that there are two forms of food in this world: primary food and secondary food. Primary food is not edible. Secondary is. The stuff on your plate that goes into your mouth is secondary food. Primary foods are the things that truly nourish you – as a whole person.

Once I understood and applied the concept of primary and secondary foods, I got back in tune with myself again. **I realized that health, nutrition and wellness is NOT all about food**. I relaxed a bit and had some vegetarian animal foods, like eggs. This lessened the feeling of restriction for me and gave me back a feeling of free will. Instantly, I reclaimed my excitement for life, got back into moving and dancing, and the rest is history.

Primary foods are the things in life that really feed us. What are the things in life that truly feed and nourish you, give you energy, and make you happy?

For me, empowering and inspiring people through communication and connection is my mission. One of my biggest challenges has been finding how I can be creative and how to express myself through my work and through my mission. **I call this self-realization (career).**

I feel energized and inspired when I connect and enjoy time with a friend, my sister or brother, my family. This primary food is my **meaningful relationships**.

I feel alive and full of energy after a workout, or a run or an aerial dance class! I can feel the sweat dripping and the energy flowing through my body. I feel alive. This primary food is my **physical activity**.

When I sit under a blossoming tree in nature or when I stop to watch the sunset, I'm reminded that I am part of something bigger than me, that life is simple (depending on your perspective). I calm down. I have a chance to catch my breath and just be. It's a feeling I wish to have more often throughout the day.

I've learned to appreciate the time I spend alone with myself. I come to understand things about myself when I stop and make time for me. It's strange, but I often feel light, positive and peaceful after spending some time alone. Getting to know myself, developing my personality, is inspiring and exciting. This primary food is my **personal growth and self-connection**.

These areas make up the four primary food pillars. When we nourish and satisfy these areas of our life, we nourish our whole being, and our focus on edible food becomes less important, or secondary.

When we neglect and "starve" ourselves of the primary foods of life, we use secondary edible foods to fill the emptiness or void.

The next time you feel hungry, ask yourself, what kind of food are you hungry for?

DO YOU LIVE TO EAT OR EAT TO LIVE?

When I hear people say, "If I can't eat steak anymore, I'd rather die," I wonder how it's possible we got ourselves to a point where our life and happiness depends on consuming a single food. If our happiness is determined by what goes on our plate, maybe we need to check our primary food balance.

Are we using secondary food to fulfill the lack of primary foods in our life?

The more balanced our primary foods are, the less we depend on secondary edible foods for emotional and mental satisfaction. When we're in balance, we can move closer to the concept that "I eat to live, to nourish my body." When we no longer need to fill empty parts of our lives, we lose our obsession with food, decrease our cravings and re-establish a healthy relationship with it. We can finally eat with the objective of nourishing our physical body with nutrient-rich foods.

|221|

SECONDARY FOODS NOURISH OUR BODIES AND PROVIDE ESSENTIAL NUTRIENTS. HOWEVER, THESE FOODS DON'T COME CLOSE TO FEEDING OUR SPIRIT THE WAY PRIMARY FOODS DO.

BALANCING PRIMARY FOODS

Most of us find that primary foods are a part of our lives, but we usually live off one or two primary foods, creating an imbalance. For example, we all know workaholics that feed off their career. Their sense of self-worth and confidence come solely from their success in their work. Take that away and they can become depressed and feel lost. These people would benefit from creating a deeper connection with themselves, finding time to reflect on their life and who they are. Perhaps getting out of their comfort zone and into a dance class! Interestingly, this will in fact benefit this person in their work with new perspectives and problem-solving capacities.

Then there are the sports fanatics. While exercise can be a healthy addiction for many people, some rely heavily on sports and exercise to escape other issues in their life or their lack of other primary foods.

Some people find that their sun and moon, their north, south, east and west, their source of energy, all comes from one other person, their relationship, and they fear it ending. Balancing the four primary foods is essential for these people. Perhaps getting into a routine of physical activity might help balance this fear. It may also improve the relationship.

RELATIONSHIPS

Friendship and romance are both forms of relationships. Healthy relationships are meaningful. They are energizing, boost our mood and bring us positivity. Do you feel vital after hanging out with your friends, family or partner? Make sure you are being energized by your relationships rather than drained. A healthy relationship is an exchange, where both individuals energize each other. If you feel drained, exhausted or low after hanging out with certain people, maybe you need to explore new positive kinds of relationships which add to your vitality. Beginning new friendships can be hard at first, but be brave. There are so many amazing people out there to meet. Create the intention to make new friends that resonate with your personality today, rather than simply hanging out with the same people because it's comfortable. We all change, and it's ever so refreshing to meet new people and have new conversations!

Many of us long to be loved and accepted by others. It's as if we have forgotten that we have an eternal fountain of love inside ourselves. Sometimes when we start a romantic relationship, the focus becomes trying to make the other person like us, or fall in love with us, and we forget to find out if, in fact, we really like them. We are seduced into the game of acceptance. However, our acceptance of ourselves is more important. A healthy relationship is one where we can share what we already foster for ourselves with another person: acceptance, love, inner peace, and the joy to be, to learn, to understand and to grow – together.

We only look to be accepted by others because we don't accept ourselves. Once we accept ourselves, we don't feel the need to be accepted by others. Self-acceptance is the gateway to self-connection. Accepting that I couldn't see, accepting my limits, was the only way that I could start to see things differently.

Once we accept ourselves, we can value ourselves and no longer need to be valued by others; we can really share the experience of a relationship without expectation.

SELF-REALIZATION/ CREATIVITY/ CAREER

One of the most successful women in business, Oprah Winfrey, says that happiness is when our actions are in alignment with our spirit. I call this self-realization.

"Don't ask yourself what the world needs; ask yourself what makes you come alive. And then go and do that. Because what the world needs is people who have come alive."
Harold Whitman

I'm reluctant to call this primary food "career". Most of us think we are doing great when we are successful and making the big bucks. I'm not talking about that kind of success because I don't agree with that concept of success.

> "Success is a lousy teacher. It seduces smart people into thinking they can't lose."
> *Bill Gates*

This primary food is about realizing and manifesting a part of yourself, your own true creativity. Sometimes you're lucky to be passionate about something and get paid for doing what you love. Sometimes the challenge is learning to love what you do. **Do what you love or learn to love what you do.**

A self-realizing career is one that gives you the chance to exercise your creativity. Every career can be creative; it's about finding the right perspective. You might love numbers; it may be connecting with people; or perhaps building things. Whatever it is, release your creativity and let it flourish. You may need to get out of your comfort zone to unlock your creativity and gain a new perspective.

Being your true self is the only requirement that actually matters. Make the best of every situation. **Bring your joy to the table every day.** If you are at a school or in a job that you don't like, take a different perspective. There might be something you do like that you hadn't noticed because your perspective kept you from seeing it. We can learn from every situation, and use our imagination to find ways to love what we do!

Do everything to the best of your ability. Sometimes we can be unhappy in a job, but it might not be because it's not the right job! If you're unhappy, it's likely you're not bringing your energy to it, or you have the wrong perspective. Sometimes when we bring our own energy to a job, we see it in a different light. Focusing on another primary food can help us gain perspective, and when we return to our "boring" job we find we have solutions we hadn't had before!

> "Act as if what you do makes a difference. It does."
> *William James*

PHYSICAL ACTIVITY

Engage in regular and fun physical activity. Our bodies are made to move, they are dying to move! It's detrimental to deprive your body of movement. Be imaginative and find ways to move that you enjoy. Once you break through the mental barrier

|224|

and lethargy, you won't know why you ever stopped moving. I like to get outside with friends or family for walks, hikes, swims. But above all, put on some music and wiggle, wiggle, wiggle!

SELF-CONNECTION – THOUGHTS, PERSONAL GROWTH AND DEVELOPMENT

Taking time to chill on your own can be miraculous (this includes no electronics at all). The silence and nothingness give space for reflection, understanding and realization, which can teach us about ourselves. Positive and creative thoughts, personal growth and awareness are central to creating a relationship with yourself. We honestly cannot have a relationship with others if we don't have one with ourselves. Get to know yourself, who you are, what you like, and spend some time alone more often than once in a while. Make a date with yourself!

Do you like yourself? Is there anything you would like to change? We are an evolving species, and can choose to evolve consciously, rather than unconsciously, and create a personality we love, which is in alignment with our essence/spirit. **True happiness and empowerment come when your personality is aligned with your spirit.**

PRIMARY FOOD AND CRAVINGS

My relationship with secondary food drastically improved once I balanced my primary foods. The why, what, when, where and how of eating became simpler, friendlier for my body.

In every first consultation, I introduce this concept to my clients. This helps us understand where the craving for or dependency on certain foods is rooted.

When a client comes for a session, we always strive to understand the underlying reason for their issues. Most of our eating habits are a reflection of our thoughts and emotions. Most of us use food as an emotional buffer, to push down thoughts and feelings we don't like dealing with.

When we talk about health and nutrition, everyone's focus is on food. But is food the real cause of our cravings and irregular eating habits? In MorLife Wellness, we make a point not to obsess about food. In fact, we dig deeper and go straight to the cause or reason WHY you are eating a certain way.

Balancing your primary foods changes your perspective from "I can't but I want to" to "I can but I don't want to".

|225|

WHAT'S YOUR PRIMARY FOOD BALANCE?

What kind of food are you craving? What kind of nourishment is missing in your life?

Try this exercise and notice what your primary food balance looks like. What part of your life would you like to improve?

The MorLife Wheel helps you reflect on your primary foods by creating a visual image of your primary food balance. The wheel shows a continuation of the kinds of things in life that feed us.

Fill in your wheel and use it to create an action plan. Here's an example:

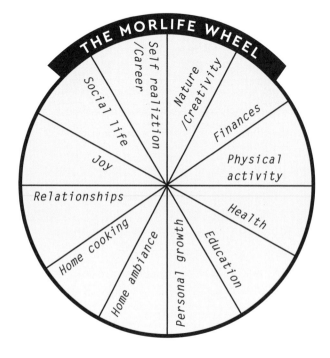

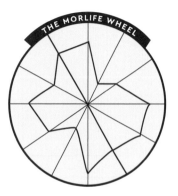

1. Rate your level of satisfaction with each area of your life by drawing a dot on the line:
   center of the wheel = 0
   outer edge = 10

2. Connect the dots to see your MorLife Wheel

3. What do you think? Are there imbalances? Determine where to spend more time and energy to create balance.

TAKE SMART ACTION

This SMART action plan will help you dedicate time and energy to the areas of your life that you have *kind of forgotten about*. Make a table with three columns. In the left column, write the specific area that you want to work on and improve, like home cooking or social life. In the middle column, write detailed SMART action steps with dates. SMART stands for Specific, Measurable, Achievable, Relevant and Time-based. For example, cook with friends (Jo and Nick) once a week on Thursdays. In the right column, record your progress and make notes.

Here are some examples and suggestions:

AREA TO IMPROVE	SMART ACTION STEP	NOTES & PROGRESS
Home cooking - cook more often at home	Start cooking two times a week at home. Invite friends for dinner and cook with them.	Prepare recipes to cook and shopping lists. Tue: Roasted veggies with tossed salad and tahini dressing Sun: Chickpea and pumpkin coconut curry
Physical Activity - move more	Start walking every Tuesday before work with Sierra.	Get gym gear ready on Monday!
Joy	Read The Power of Now by Eckart Tolle Subscribe to the MorLife Wellness programme	Bought the book! Subscribed to MLW programme
Improve finances	Begin saving £20 per month (no amount is too little to start with)	Done

Carolina's story

Balancing primary foods was a real challenge at first, especially living in this accelerated modern world. Seeing the different areas of my life laid out on the MorLife wheel was very clarifying - how some areas were totally taking priority over others, and funnily enough I was not aware of it!! Small juggles and shifts in my everyday life (like walking 20 mins a day, making space for a drink with a friend once every two weeks, allowing myself spiritual time in nature to reconnect in between hectic daily schedules or taking a long look at my home environment and adjusting it as best as possible) really changed my health, my weight (I lost 10kg) and above all, I feel alive again!

Carolina, age 35, Homeopathic Physician and single mother

TAKING IT TO THE NEXT LEVEL

Now we can look at what we might want to add rather than which area we need to work on. You could be satisfied with your primary food areas but there are always ways to improve them.

Take your Action Plan to the next level by creating objectives in every primary food area of your life.

Physical activity goals:
Relationship goals:
Self-realization and career goals:
Self-connection and self-care goals:

Be creative and write down anything that comes to mind! Remember that trying new things is a great way to get out of your head and, according to neuroscience, will only make you more intelligent!

Writing your wishes and objectives down with your own hand is the first step to manifestation. When we make ourselves accountable, things can shift on every level.

Get out of your comfort zone

If you feel like you need more joy in your life, start a dance class this week, even if you think you don't know how to dance! Getting out of your comfort zone puts you in the now and will change your life! It gets you out of your head! In fact, research confirms that learning something new, like dancing, and having to make acute instant decisions is highly beneficial for the brain and helps prevent mental diseases such as dementia, Alzheimer's and Parkinson's.

Can getting out of your comfort zone make you more intelligent?

Placing yourself out of your comfort zone, in a brand-new environment, engages the frontal association cortex and hippocampus, regions of the brain that are linked to intelligence and "higher order executive" functions such as planning, decision making and problem solving. Stimulating this part of the brain by courageously trying new activities will improve your cognitive acuity and capacity to respond creatively when problems or challenges arise in any area of your life. These activities create new neural pathways which are fundamental to our brain's health.

"Our brain constantly rewires its neural pathways, as needed. If it doesn't need to, then it won't."

Dr Joseph Coyle, Harvard Medical School psychiatrist

So make sure you are trying something new and getting out of your cosy comfort zone every week! Salsa, dancehall, or saxophone classes... which is it gonna be?

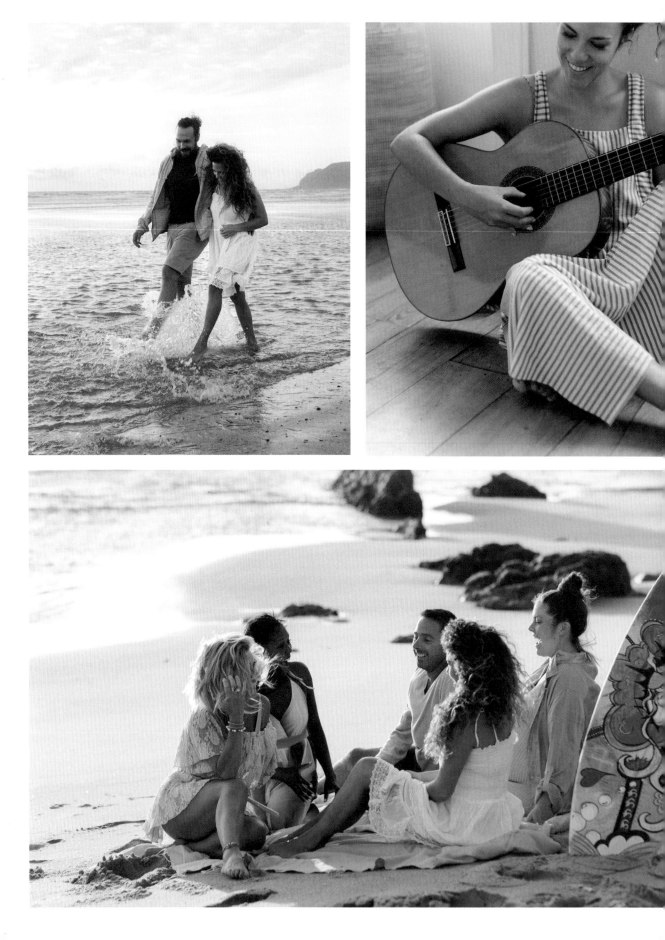

Three ways to get high naturally

Here are three ways to increase your vibration to help you develop all four primary food areas.

1. **Be courageous and shine as bright as you really are.**

2. **Emotions are e-motion.** They are there to help us create motion. Use emotions to inspire, move, and change you. Instead of staying irritated, frustrated, angry, sad or depressed, find out what brought on this emotion and create a baby-step action plan. Negative emotions like irritation, anger and frustration are self-destructive and serve no purpose other than to help us blame others.

3. **Avoid thoughts with words like "never", "should" and "can't".** They create chemicals in the body that weaken our physiology. No wonder we're exhausted at the end of the day! Recognize and change a negative or limiting thought. For example, change "I can't meet this deadline," to "I don't know how I'm going to meet this deadline." The chemicals produced by the body as a response to this kind of thought are more likely to support you in fulfilling your goal.

**Reset your mindset, make it a new era, and take these
three thoughts with you!**

|231|

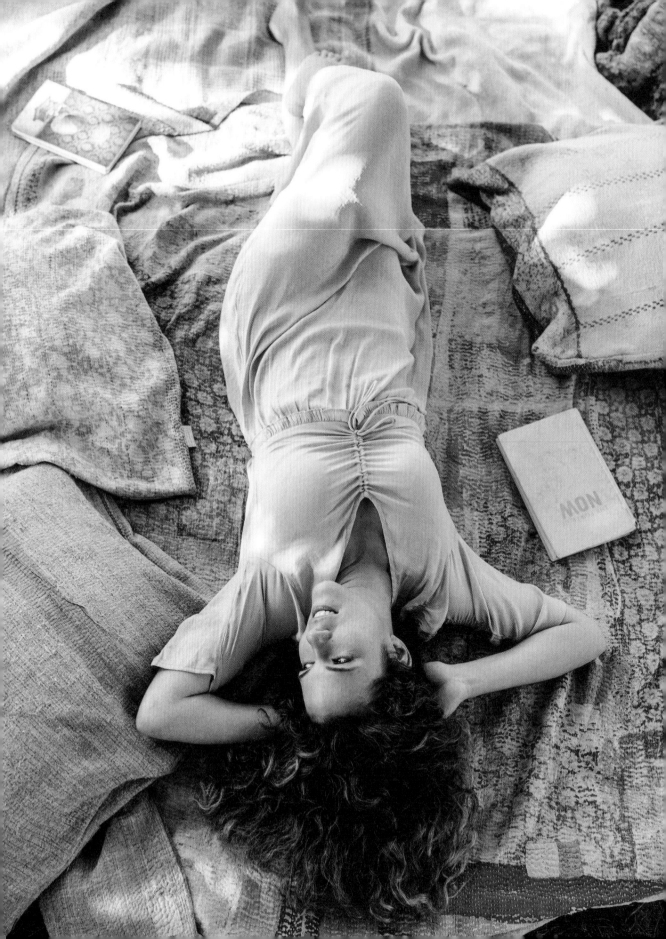

> *"Can you remember who you were, before the world told you who you should be?"*
> Charles Bukowski

Chapter 13

YOU ARE WHAT YOU ~~EAT~~ THINK

YOU DA BOSS!

HOW GOOD YOUR LIFE FEELS IS UP TO YOU. IT IS WITHIN YOUR CONTROL. IT'S NOT HOW GOOD YOU ARE, BUT HOW GOOD YOU WANT TO BE. ALL OF US ARE PRESENTED WITH THE TOOLS WE NEED TO CREATE A LIFE WE TRULY ENJOY AND LOVE. SO, WHAT IS HOLDING US BACK?

Your thoughts and emotions can have a stronger effect on your health than what you eat. You can eat all the right foods, avoid the baddies and remove the toxins, but if you have your thoughts in the wrong place, you ain't got nothing. Thoughts are the foundation of a stable, joyful, healthy life.

Your thoughts or words can affect your physiology in a negative or positive way. Research has shown how thoughts become biology, and how repeated negative thoughts can lead to a number of problems like fibromyalgia, muscle pain, fatigue, tiredness, obesity, cancer, indigestion, acid reflux, heart burn, heart attacks and more.

The negative emotions of anger, fear and resentment can be the most powerful and acidifying of all emotions.

Positive feelings actually make the body more alkaline and strengthen the immune system!

People have thought attacks, not heart attacks. There are published studies showing that over 80 per cent of all heart attacks are emotionally triggered. Experts say that people don't die of a heart attack, they die of a thought attack, which leads to the heart attack.

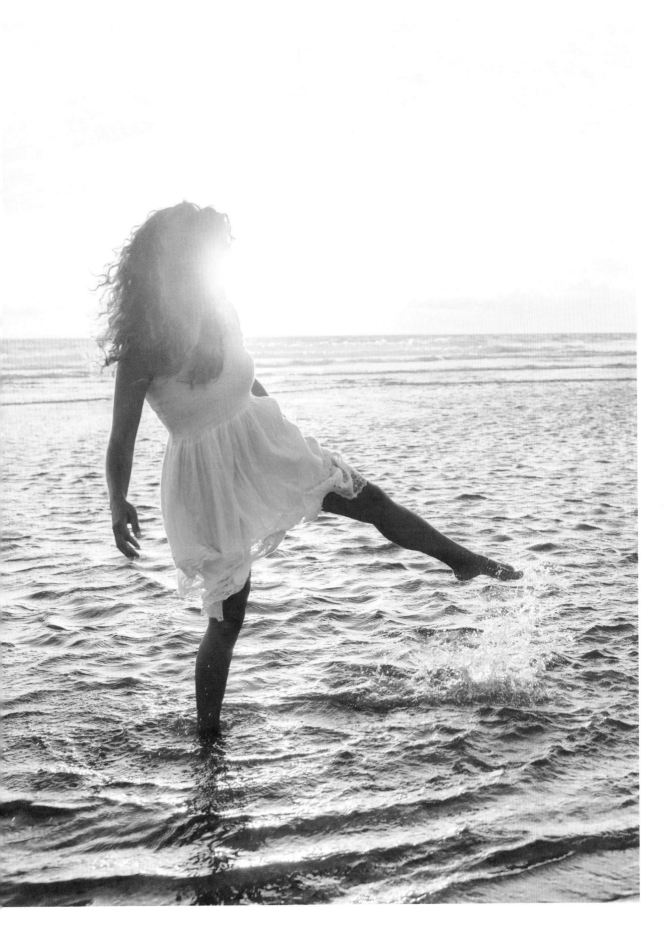

THE POWER OF THOUGHTS

"Watch your thoughts;
they become words.
Watch your words;
they become actions.
Watch your actions;
they become habits.
Watch your habits;
they become your
character.
Watch your character;
it becomes your
destiny."

Anonymous

The Japanese scientist, Dr Masaru Emoto, has shown that our thoughts also influence the world around us. Dr Emoto photographed frozen samples of polluted water before and after prayer was performed over the water, and distilled water before and after exposure to music, such as heavy metal and Beethoven. He also taped words to jars of distilled water like, "You make me sick. I will kill you," and "Love and appreciation."

The energy from positive words and thoughts, even if only written, created exquisite snowflake-like patterns in the water. The less positive words created dark, grey images showing disorder and toxicity. Our bodies are 70 per cent water. Imagine how our daily thoughts affect the water molecules inside of us! Imagine that our thoughts don't only affect our water molecules, but can even affect those around us!

WHAT'S STOPPING YOU FROM BEING BRILLIANT?

Marianne Williamson, author and lecturer says, "Our deepest fear is not that we are inadequate. Our deepest fear is that we are powerful beyond measure." It is our light, not our darkness, that most frightens us. We ask ourselves, "Who am I to be brilliant, gorgeous, talented and fabulous?" Actually, who are you not to be? Playing small does not serve the world. There is nothing enlightened about shrinking so that others will not feel insecure around you. We are all meant to shine, as children do. **We were born to manifest the light that is within us. As we let our own light shine bright, we unconsciously inspire others to do the same. So, what's stopping you from shining bright?**

Having a positive attitude does change the experience and outcome of our life. We actually create energizing chemicals in our brains when we have positive thoughts. This triggers confidence and joy, and subsequently attracts positive people, situations and much more. You may not believe this but I have so many stories to prove this is true.

From feeling joy for no apparent reason to feeling happy and full of life, from increasing our confidence and literally strengthening our body to prevent illness – thoughts are the foundation of wellness and vitality.

MorLife Wellness is not a diet, nor is it a lifestyle. It is a mindset, a way of thinking that will create the perfect resources for you to build the life you choose from the inside out – based on empowerment rather than external power. Your mindset is the foundation that everything is built on. When we have a healthy soil, any amazing plant or dream can be nurtured and grown. Similarly, when we have a fertile, positive mindset, and we are prepared to trust, receive and co-exist with nature, we can create a life beyond what we can imagine. Your

spirit is the seed – if your mindset is negative and contaminated, your spirit won't manifest its essence into a life of full potential.

"The world as we have created it is a process of our thinking. It cannot be changed without changing our thinking."
Albert Einstein

|237|

POSITIVE THINKING

We've all heard the story of Aunt Janie, who ate all she wanted, smoked, drank and did it all, but she was always happy, dancing, loving the world, and lived to the ripe old age of 103. Her vitality was connected to her positivity.

Visualizing positive images, being optimistic, striving to see the lesson and grow from every situation, even when it's miserable, making an effort to smile inside, or be kind, all of these are examples of manifesting a positive mindset; it's an uplifting way of life that creates energy rather than draining energy. However big the problem, positivity is always a more fun ride than negativity.

FAKE IT TILL YOU MAKE IT

We create unnecessary suffering and negativity for ourselves. Life is an unexpected succession of lessons that have to be lived to be understood. There are moments of ease and many challenges, but in general life is the flavour that you choose. In comparison to most of the chapters in this book where we need to pace ourselves and take small steps, when it comes to the mind, it's quite different. Often it's necessary and important to push through the initial resistance. Faking it until we make it is about creating new neurological pathways that bring more into our life rather than limit it. Pretending to be happy, positive and excited about your life is a perfect place to start if you are not feeling this way. **The better you fake it, the more real it becomes!**

Most of us are naturally self-destructive. It's easy to surrender to this part of us, but this means we are choosing to extinguish our own light.

We live in a world controlled by thoughts. Do you ever feel like you are a prisoner to your thoughts? Real freedom comes with the capacity to detach from them. In fact, maybe the unpleasant thought you're experiencing isn't even yours. Perhaps it has been borrowed from someone else and instilled into your subconscious.

BECOMING AWARE OF OUR THOUGHTS

What's it like when we start watching our thoughts, observing them as an outsider, not being led by them? Did you know that, on average, humans have 70,000 thoughts a day? That's about fifty per minute. How conscious and aware are we about the thoughts we are having? Are they original thoughts and are they ours? Are they uplifting and positive or draining and self-defeating? Do these thoughts influence important decisions and are they steering us in a particular direction? Are we in control of our journey?

Positive thoughts boost our mood and can create good energy. Negative thoughts do the opposite. They create a domino effect of destructive energy. It's incredible how my mood sets the tone for my day, and when I'm irritated, frustrating things happen to me – my tyre bursts or the internet stops working. How do we stop our thoughts from taking over, repeating the record, day after day?

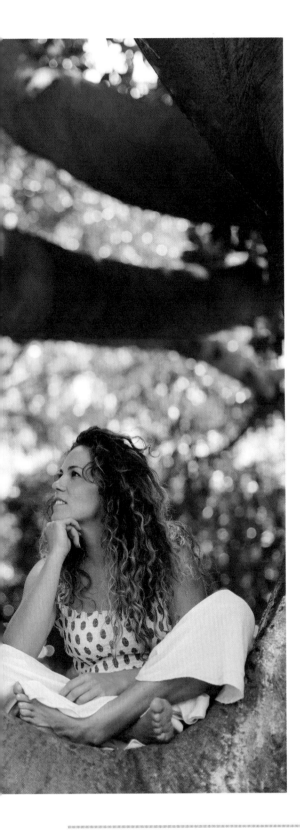

Get out of your own way

I have spent more than half of my life trying to understand the concept of health, vitality, beauty, happiness and joy. Food is important. It's important to know about it so that you can stop intoxicating yourself and avoid ingesting artificial substances or GM food that harms your body. But food is pretty straightforward. For me, the hardest thing was accepting that my mindset and thoughts were limiting my life. We can be as healthy as we want, but if we don't believe in or like ourselves, if we don't create a relationship with ourselves, we won't find fulfilment, joy and everything we are looking for.

|239|

TWO TYPES OF THOUGHTS

Because thoughts are intangible, it can be confusing to talk about them. I've defined two types of thoughts categorized by their origin. This can help us recognize original thoughts from ones that don't truly belong to us.

1. CONDITIONED THINKING:

Conditioned thoughts can be described as thoughts derived from society, culture, education, ancestral family patterns and what has been projected onto us by others, hence, the origin of these thoughts are not ours. These thoughts are conditioned by the external world and projected onto our inside world. How healthy these thoughts are is debatable.

For example: "I should be married by now; I'm such a failure" is not an original thought. It is a conditioned thought, imbedded into our mindset from childhood. "I haven't found true love; I'm not worthy." These thoughts are what our culture has educated us to expect. If you think about it, girls play with baby dolls from a very early age; they are inherently being educated that their value comes

from becoming a mother. However, this value is external; it should be a woman's calling, not so that she can be valued by society.

These forms of thinking happen in our mind. Most of our thoughts are negative. The viscous cycle of negative thoughts is easier to surrender to than making the effort to think positively. There are many arguments of why this is, but I like to simplify: we all have a destructive programming that simply needs to be recognized, disarmed and dismantled.

2. CREATIVE THINKING:

A creative thought is one that is unique to you. One that comes from you, before you were bombarded with the ideals of society. A thought that comes from your essence, your higher self. A thought that brings insight to who you truly are so you can evolve consciously.

Why do children always ask "Why?", "How come?" They come from a place of discovery, simplicity, humility and yearning to understand why and how. When did we stop

|240|

asking these questions of ourselves? We could call this a creative or reflective thought, with the intention of insight or understanding ourselves better. For example, you might ask yourself, "Why did I get so angry there?" or, "What is it about her that irritates me? Maybe I wish I could be as confident as she is." "Why do I crave chocolate every day at five p.m.?" "What is my intention with my actions and choices?" Asking ourselves the right question, which leads to another question, reflection and perspective, is a creative thought process. Let's challenge ourselves through questioning our nature, intentions and attitudes, by asking, "Why?"

YOU CAN ONLY CHANGE YOURSELF

As a young enthusiast wanting to change the world, I was sad to hear one of my great teachers tell me this. We cannot change others; we can perhaps inspire other people, but really, we have little influence on others. When I was a child and teenager, in any difficult situation with friends or boys, my mum always turned the picture back on to me. How could I grow and learn from this situation rather than focus on or blame others? I adopted this approach in life. In every situation, there is always something to learn

by asking ourselves why, what and how. It's not always a simple approach. When we are upset it's easier and more fulfilling in that moment to blame others. But, in fact, it's quite incredible what we can discover when we use every opportunity to understand why we attract certain situations and what we can learn from them.

Creative thinking happens when we are in the present moment, when we stop paying attention to our mind, when we allow space for nothingness. This is where magic happens, when scientists have epiphanies; Einstein made most of his discoveries when he was in between his logical thoughts.

The painter Dali captured his creativity between conscious and unconscious states. He would fall asleep with a spoon in his hand, so that as he fell asleep the spoon would drop onto the floor and wake him up. In this in-between state, he would paint.

CREATIVE THINKING CAN HELP US EVOLVE

When we question our actions, our behaviours, our intentions, we challenge our mindset which can filter and disarm negative programming and patterns. When we find ourselves in repetitive unpleasant situations, we can be sure that something within has to change so that we can attract something different, something better. Creative thinking and questioning yourself creates space for creative solutions, "aha" moments. It unlocks your own fountain of wisdom that exists within your higher self. This, simply put, is consciousness and awareness.

Questioning your everyday thoughts, actions and intentions can help you understand yourself better. For example, perhaps someone irritates you. This person dresses nicely and is always smiling. You find them fake and annoying. Questioning why they irritate you can help you gain insight about your own wishes in life. Would you like to care better for yourself? Is it hard for you to find time to be positive and feel happy? Would you like to feel beautiful? Sometimes we judge others because we have a secret wish to be like them. Not specifically like them, but we wish to have the courage to dare to be ourselves.

Another example is judging ourselves for not eating healthier and then judging others that do make the effort to be healthy. Have you even teased or been teased by friends for making healthier lifestyle choices? By questioning our thoughts, we may find out that we do want to be different, to live differently. Or we might find we have new values, and what we used to think of as crucial is no longer important. Our perspective of life is simplified, our self-connection is boosted. Most of us are so caught up in the rat race that we don't even know what we want. Investing time in questioning ourselves and having honest, inner conversations can help us find out if the intention behind our actions and thoughts is in alignment with our higher self, who we essentially really are.

IF YOU DON'T KNOW WHO YOU ARE, IT'S HARD TO BE YOU

Through this process, I discovered numerous times that my thoughts came from a feeling of lack, a sense of fear. When I became aware of the origin of the thought, I could let it go, and connect with my own strength and source of passion for life. This moment – which many call an "aha" moment – changes your experience every day so that you begin to create a personality and a life that you truly love and enjoy, a personality that is aligned with your spirit.

The thing about consciousness is you can't go back. Your life changes forever.

DETACHMENT: THE FIRST STEP TO CREATIVE THINKING

It's time to become aware of our own thoughts. Are our thoughts original, unique, creative? Or are they conditioned? Buddha talks about the capacity to watch our own thoughts and emotions as an observer with detachment. Step outside of your ego, the concept of "me", and just be an observer of yourself. Question your thinking and thought patterns. Ask yourself where your thoughts come from.

When we are able to detach from our thoughts, we realize that we are not one with them, and therefore have a choice to either listen to them or not. For example, "What if they don't like me?" is a thought, not an absolute reality. It comes from a place of fear and lacking. If your mindset believes that you are your thoughts, then you are attached to them. In fact, the ideal is that you understand that your thoughts are not you. We must be able to detach from our thoughts and observe them as an entirely separate entity – and even check that they are in tune with what we wish for ourselves, not seeds that were planted in our mindset by others that influenced our lives. When you are attached to your thoughts, you are not free

from them. If you can detach from them, simply observe them and even shoo the negative ones away, you begin to live more freely. This way it becomes easier to connect and be aware of the subtle presence of the essence of the real you, the higher source of yourself (your spirit). You are now conscious and can make space for conscious thinking, living and evolving.

A HUMAN WITHOUT CONSCIOUSNESS OR AWARENESS IS NOTHING MORE THAN A ROBOT

Many of us live our lives on autopilot, not really experiencing ourselves in the world around us. As kids, from the moment we can speak, we are told to listen to others. We are told how to live, eat, rest, play, what to study, when to marry and reproduce. It's all mapped out for us. But who makes these rules?

Life is an immediate experience of connection, awareness and essence. If we are disconnected from our true self, our higher self, can we really say we are living? If we are unconsciously living, perhaps we are living a life that someone else programmed for us. What about creating our own life, our unique path, a conscious one,

|243|

that expresses who WE truly are from the inside out? When do we wake up to ourselves?

The path you take in life is yours to choose and create. If you don't choose, someone else will choose for you. What a waste of a ride! If you choose to live unconsciously, you evolve unconsciously. If you choose consciously, you evolve consciously.

Yuval Harari, a great historian who studies humankind (and author of one of my fave books *21 Lessons for the 21st Century*!) asks the question, "Are humans happier now than they were 100 years ago?" He explains clearly how culture was created by men no smarter than us. Perhaps it's time we reshape our own culture into something that is more in tune with us and nature; becoming who we're meant to be on our journey.

A SEED IS NOT A TREE – EMBRACING POSITIVE STRESS

You are fantastic. But if you don't think you are fantastic, you will never be fantastic. I've met so many wonderful, amazing, super people on my crazy journey on this planet, and so often I meet people that are unaware of how amazing they are. Our potential is always there, whether we choose and dare to realize our true self is a choice we have to make every moment, every day.

Just like a seed has the potential to grow into a tree, if it doesn't decide to sprout and begin growing, it could well remain a seed forever. The act of sprouting is highly stressful for the seed. It's like a rubber band that gets stretched and stressed, and once you let go of one side, it flies so far you lose sight of it. I call this kind of stress "positive stress" – a form of stress that makes us grow, sprout and evolve. It is necessary for personal growth and development. It can be tough, but when embraced, it unlocks the flow of life. Writing this book was one of the biggest stresses I've ever had. I had to stress myself to get it done, focus and dedicate. But once you fine-tune your physical, mental and emotional energy, and any other energy you have, into one objective, it's rather amazing what the result can be. Remember, I wrote this book with very little eyesight, a book I cannot read in print.

If I had turned my back on all the challenges, difficulties and obstacles that life presented me with as I lost my vision a little more each time; if I had given up university because I couldn't read the medical books and found it ever so frustrating to trust and believe that I would find a solution; if I didn't dig deep to find courage and transform this uncomfortable stress into a positive stress, I would not feel the joy I feel and live today.

BREAKING FREE FROM OUR LIMITING THOUGHTS

In India, when an elephant is born, they tie it to a tree with a big, heavy metal chain. It tugs and tries to pull away but cannot, because it's not big and strong enough. As the elephant gets bigger, they replace the large metal chain with a smaller, lighter one. When the elephant reaches its adult size and is big and strong, they replace the chain with a thin, itty bitty rope. The elephant is strong enough to break the rope and can break free now that he's big and strong, but he does not tug or even try to get away because he thinks he cannot. He tried a few times before and his mind is set that he cannot.

We come into this world with endless creativity and intuition. As we begin to express ourselves through movement and speech, we are controlled and conditioned. Our imagination, our creativity, and our intuitive voice shuts down as our mindset is moulded and limited by society. Just like the elephant, we have the strength to break the rope that holds us from being free, yet our mindset is so well embedded that we don't believe it's possible.

If we are able to detach from the situation and observe ourselves like we can observe and imagine a huge, powerful elephant feeling prisoner to the rope, we are creating consciousness. This awareness creates space for a solution that breaks you free from your limiting thoughts and mindset.

The fact that I couldn't see placed me into a mindset that I was less, that I was inferior. I decided I was not going to stay in this place and I decided I was going to take myself and my condition less seriously. I was going to be silly, vulnerable and even feel super uncomfortable at times. What I was not going to do was stay quiet and simply suffer with fear of being judged. I made my vulnerability my strength. I decided I would share my reality with joy and fun. Make it something interesting, rather than having people feel sorry for me. I am no victim; I simply have a different vision of life. "I don't see so well, but I see much more than many people, I soon found out." Just because we have ears doesn't mean we listen; just because we have eyes doesn't mean we look. My attitude toward my limitations created opportunities and taught me how to make the best of every situation.

My friend, Vanda, chose a life that had little guarantees. She followed her passion, her intuition, her creative thoughts, not her fears. In fact, she connected to her fears, detached from them to motivate and help her grow and become an internationally renowned professional dancer and choreographer. She says, "Follow your passion, create your own identity and path. Even if it means you're not going to see your friends and family on the weekends. Don't take what people tell you too seriously. People believe in you if you believe in yourself! If my parents hadn't told me to listen to myself, and if I hadn't given up certain social pleasures back then, I would never have got to be where I am today. So, continue to believe in yourself, because people eventually will too!"

CHOOSE JOY

Joy is the ultimate vibration of life. However, what most of us don't realize until much later in life is that joy comes only from inside. **You cannot buy, arrange for, reserve, or wear joy.** It is the essence of our being, and without it, we're not really living.

Find out who you are, where you come from, and where you're going. Life is a long time. Take one step at a time. Be gentle, kind and joyful.

Carolina's story

Carolina moved alone to a new country to study for her degree in psychology. After graduating, she got a day job as a psychologist but things didn't feel right. After reflection, she realized she wanted to share her musical talents. But it wasn't going to be an easy road. All the effort she had invested into getting through university: would she have the courage to let all that go?
"In my journey with music over the last nine years I've learned that the quiet voice within speaks from a place of love, connection and truth. I believe it will always guide you toward what will make you happy."

Carolina is now a successful singer and producer.

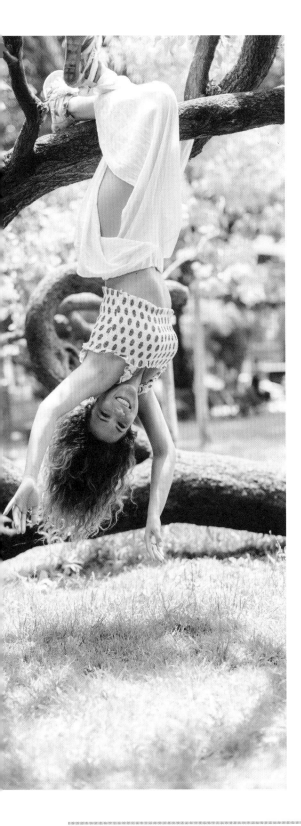

CHANGE YOUR PERSPECTIVE

"We do not experience things as they really are! We experience things only through a filter and that filter determines what information will enter our awareness and what will be rejected. If we change the filter (our belief/thought system), then we automatically experience the world in a completely different way."

David Wolfe, health expert and author

10 Ways to Refresh Your Perspective

1. **Be grateful.** The grass is greener on THIS side! Create a gratitude journal. Write down five things you're grateful for every night. We get caught up in life and forget what we have. Even when we think we don't have it all, appreciating who we are and what we have puts things into perspective. Do this every night for two weeks. Try not to repeat things. You may find your life is much better than you thought!

2. **Move.** Motion beats meditation. You won't move forward until you move out of your own way. Moving takes us out of our head and into our body and breath. Challenging and new movement is the best way to keep your attention focused in the present moment, and away from past or future thoughts and emotions. Try a dance or Pilates class, swimming or horse riding – anything where you can't think about your life because you're too busy having fun.

3. **Eliminate mental toxins.** Stop and ignore negative inner chatter. Don't take yourself too seriously. When you hear negative thoughts, throw them out, delete, cancel and restart. Try imagining your favourite place, sing a song, replace the negative thought with a positive statement. Becoming aware that you are having a negative thought is the coolest thing ever. You have made the hardest step – now all you have to do is detach from it, realize it's not a useful thought. Thank it, and say, "I don't need you now." Try to understand where it comes from and focus your attention on something that you do want. When good things happen to us, we often allow negative thoughts to doubt that we deserve it. For example, getting promoted. Reminding yourself why you're good at your job and why you love it can help to counteract those thoughts. Focus your intentions on the positives. Remind yourself that everything new is challenging; it's part of finding humility in yourself. Thank yourself for having the courage to try something new and be open to the discoveries that this adventure could bring. Laugh at yourself rather than judge yourself. You are daring and cool for getting out of your comfort zone. Just relax and enjoy the discomfort of not knowing. When you feel the negativity arise in your head, remind yourself of all the things you are grateful for and how you are doing the best that you can.

4. **Throw out limiting thoughts and beliefs.** Deconstruct beliefs that no longer serve you. Whoever invented that belief was no smarter than you. For example, you should earn more money, you should be married by now, you should do this or that. You can build and create your own values and goals. Ask yourself what you would like, and create goals from there.

5. **Surround yourself with positive people.** When we get stuck in a negative spiral, sometimes it's helpful to speak to someone that can give us perspective and won't feed our negative thoughts. Find positive people to surround yourself with, even if it's just one person.

6. **Let go of resistance.** "If you change nothing, nothing will change," or, "Nothing changes IF nothing changes." Or, like Albert Einstein said, "If you always do what you always did, then you will always get what you always got." If we want different results, we need to do something different. Make small changes. Find your unique rhythm and push past resistance at your own pace.

7. **Reflect and analyse what went wrong.** There are no mistakes, only lessons. Lessons will repeat to you in various forms until you have learned them. See every experience as an opportunity to learn, understand and grow. I ask myself how I got into a situation, what part of me attracted this moment, and what I can work on to improve myself.

8. **Don't play the victim.** We create our own lives. It's our responsibility. If you don't like where you are, change it. You are not a tree. There is always a solution; be creative and you'll surprise yourself. I always have the choice to make change happen if I want to. What you make of your life is up to you.

9. **Compare yourself to yourself.** Comparing ourselves to others discards everything we've created in our own lives. It's easy to want what others have. Instead, use them as inspiration and motivation to create your life. Find the value in everything you have experienced.

10. **Help someone else.** Taking the focus off ourselves can change our perspective on life. It gives us a chance to get out of our heads and to realize that perhaps we're looking at our own situation in the wrong way. Sometimes we make more of an effort to be positive for others than we do for ourselves. Help a friend or colleague or go to a shelter or institution and help those in need (this also helps tip one).

EMOTIONS – USE THEM TO EVOLVE

"Once you become aware of what stands in your way and become willing to release it, you signal to the universe that you are ready to manifest the life you were meant to live."

Cherie Carter-Scott, author of If Life Is a Game, These Are the Rules

E-motion is energy in motion. Energy that has come to our attention to help us change or move something. The word comes from the Latin emovere, meaning "to disturb".

The trick is to use the emotion you feel to take action, rather than becoming the emotion. For example, anger can help us understand that we don't agree with a specific situation.

This can help us address and communicate how we feel, without emotion. Through communication we can learn compassion, get insight and either change the situation or learn to accept new situations.

Many of us, however, become the emotion and often get stuck in it. Becoming our emotions keeps us in the past or future – we become frozen. This does not help us take steps or develop our personality. Don't discard your emotions. Use them like signals to help you make choices and take action. Learn to communicate without emotions. For example, "What happened yesterday made me feel rejected. I felt hurt. I felt uncomfortable." Rather than, "You hurt me. You didn't listen to me." I suggest that we communicate when we no longer feel emotional; waiting a day or longer helps us detach from the negative emotion.

Taking it further and reflecting on our emotions helps us learn what triggers them. This can be very useful in creating positive relationships.

DARE TO BE CHALLENGED

Every event in life occurs to teach us something about ourselves. When you feel challenged, there is always an opportunity to learn and grow. Find a moment to stop your mind and breathe. Listen to your breath, to the birds, or the cars. Scan your body from your toes to your head and find out what is uncomfortable. Is there a solution that brings relief? Do you need to make a change that scares you? Are you lost, and need to spend more time alone? Try to connect to your physical body without your mind interfering. Life is an adventure, and one of the most fun experiences is finding the answers within yourself. We cannot control every outcome, but we can control our own actions. Wait for the answers patiently. There is always an opportunity to learn and grow. This is one of the most fulfilling experiences for me. Getting through a challenging time, learning and evolving, is truly a fascinating experience.

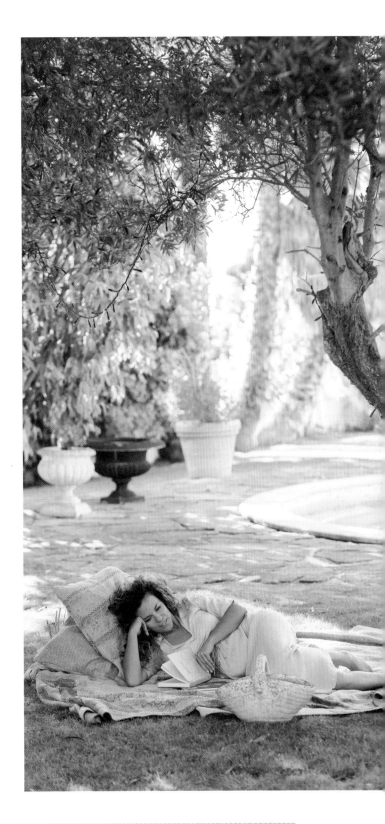

YOU ARE A SUPERHERO

"We're all born with immense natural talents, but by the time we've been through education, far too many of us have lost touch with them. Many talented, brilliant people think they're not (brilliant) because the thing they were good at in school wasn't valued or was actually stigmatized. These consequences are disastrous for individuals and for the health of our communities."

Ken Robinson, author of Creative Schools

My perspective is that we are all superstars. We need courage and willingness to discover our super power, and then accept it, instead of desiring a different one. We are great and capable of just about anything. We need to be aware of the war inside of us, between our creative and destructive thoughts. When I was sixteen years old, I was travelling alone in Hawaii and stumbled upon this little book, called *Practising the Power of Now* by Eckart Tolle. The book made me aware of my thoughts, my patterns, and how I stood in the way of myself.

As I mentioned in the beginning of this chapter, we can try every diet on the block, but if we don't change our perspective – our mind – we will always come back home to our old habits. The only way to make a change is to really get to the bottom of it all and control our mind, rather than have it control us.

I'm always thinking, and it's so hard to just stop. I think, I overthink, until I realize that I'm driving myself crazy by thinking, and then I can stop. My goal is to catch myself before I start on that rollercoaster of thoughts.

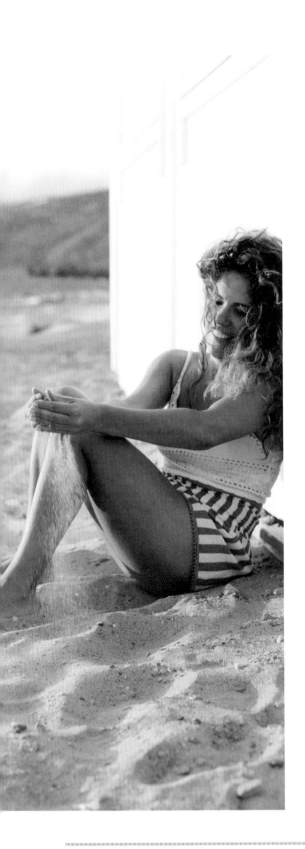

Since I'm able to catch my thoughts before they are controlling me, I'm more joyful, more positive, more productive in my life, and more proactive in achieving my goals. When I manage to get a hold on my mind, it's bliss. I've been working toward controlling my mind for many years now. It's not easy. It's like we have a programme inside us that's there for self-destruction, waiting to be triggered. Naming our triggers is a great way to become conscious and detach from them.

MAKING THE CHOICE TO CHANGE

"All great changes are preceded by chaos."
Deepak Chopra

Sometimes it can feel as if the universe is testing your level of willingness to get through every obstacle. Things seem to get harder before the ocean calms down and starts to flow.

I hope this chapter is to you what that little book I discovered in Hawaii was for me. I hope it wakes you up to yourself, makes you aware of the nature of your thoughts so that you can lead your thoughts, rather than them blindly leading you.

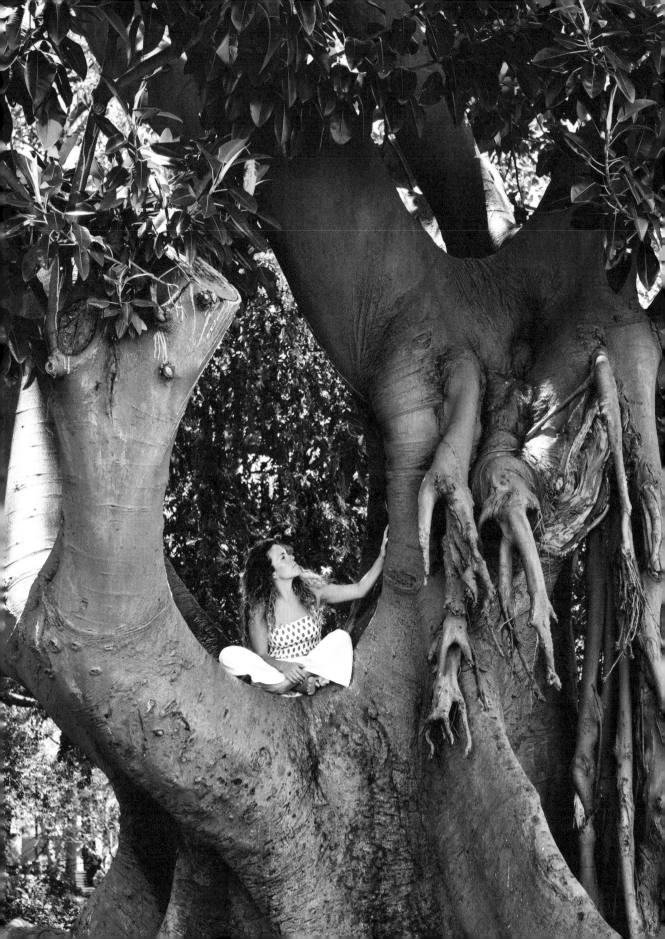

*I was in awe;
how could
Ayurveda know
me better than
I knew myself?*

Chapter 14

ROCK ANCIENT
AYURVEDIC WISDOM

LOOKING BACK TO GO FORWARD

ANCIENT INDIAN MEDICINE, THE OLDEST DOCUMENTED IN HISTORY, IS CONSIDERED TO BE THE MOTHER OF MEDICINE.

Ayurveda holds great secrets on how to stay healthy and happy for life. With a modern touch, this ancient wisdom rocks! Air, water, fire, earth or space, find out which is your predominant dosha element and how food and the external environment influence your body, mind and life!

How to pronounce it: Ah-yoor – veda

Ayurveda originated in the Himalayas, and its secrets were recorded in scriptures from 10,000–500BC! The concepts of Ayurveda are prehistoric, yet scientific and innovative. They are built upon a basic understanding of nature and life, which makes them simple and applicable to anyone. India is one of the few countries today that offers its traditional ancient medicine alongside conventional medicine. Why? Because Ayurveda works. Its approach is applied in thousands of hospitals around the world.

What makes Ayurveda simple is the fundamental concept that every cell in the universe is composed of a combination of the five great elements: ether, air, fire, water and earth. Every cell contains each of the five elements, however one or two may be more predominant. We perceive these elements through our senses, while we are also made up of the same elements. For example, muscle tissue is predominantly earth and water.

Ayurveda emphasizes the concept of balance, through which changes occur naturally. **Health and illness are underlined by balance and imbalance, which lead to comfort and discomfort, happiness and misery, respectively.** Balancing your dietary habits will effortlessly lead to subtle positive changes in your life.

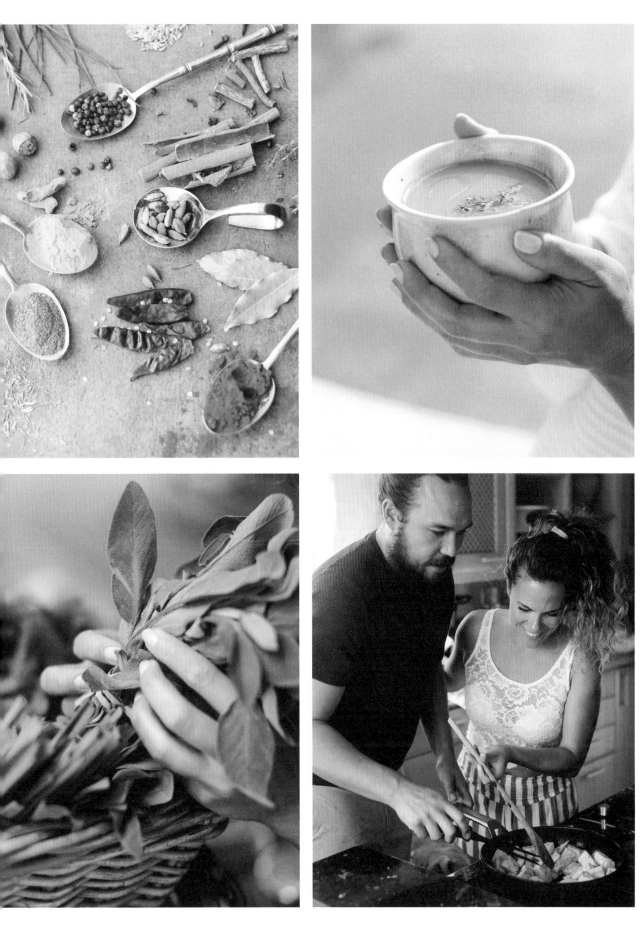

ANCIENT WISDOM ROCKS

Ayurveda is a Sanskrit word meaning "knowledge of life". It focuses on prevention of discomfort, disease and imbalance, and the body's natural ability to heal itself.

Ayurveda acknowledges that all of life, human, animal, or plant, must live in harmony with nature in order to survive (yeah!).

Ayurveda has led me to knowledge that allows me to see and understand life from a point of view that answers so many questions.

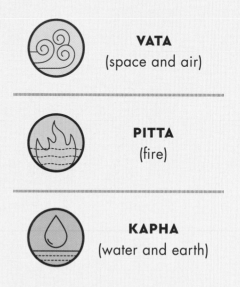

VATA
(space and air)

PITTA
(fire)

KAPHA
(water and earth)

AYURVEDA IS THE SCIENCE OF LIFE

Ayurveda is a science that takes the whole person into consideration – body, mind and spirit. It is holistic and shows how every part of the body is inherently connected. Our thoughts and emotions can affect our digestion, as our physical sensations can affect our mind.

Everything in the universe is made up of the five great elements, which exist inside and outside of our bodies. Inside the body, the five elements are represented through three doshas: vata, pitta and kapha.

Although we are made up of all five elements, we are usually dominant in one or two doshas. **The concept of the doshas is the coolest thing that exists.** They represent the whole of us: mental disposition, emotional patterns, physical appearance, and all imbalances respectively. In other words, doshas are a gateway to understanding yourself. It really rocks! People always ask me how I know things about them, like that they are naturally nervous or that they have dry skin or constipation – it's all in the wisdom of Ayurveda!

WHAT'S YOUR DOSHA?

Because we are naturally dominant in one or two doshas, we might be dominantly made up of more fire (pitta), water and earth (kapha), or space and air (vata). Just as each element has its characteristics, so do we. The beauty of Ayurvedic science is that it appreciates that no one is the same. You and I are unique, and that's perfect! Find out what makes your perfect.

Use the tables on the following pages to understand yourself better, make smarter choices for your unique dosha according to the season or even microclimate! For example, enjoy cold foods like ice cream and yoghurt (non-dairy of course!), salads and fresh fruit in the summer, when they help to cool the body down. In the winter, we are naturally attracted to warm soup that heats the body. In other words, if there is increased fire and heat outside, eat foods that are cooling and refreshing. When the external environment is cold and wet, eat warming and drying foods.

NATURE NATURALLY GROWS SPECIFIC FOODS IN EACH SEASON TO BALANCE THE ELEMENTS WITHIN OUR BODY WITH EXTERNAL ONES.

The guides on the following pages show the practical manifestation of these elements: physical, mental, emotional characteristics, including positive or unbalanced emotions. Which characteristics do you recognize?

If you want more help identifying your dosha, why not take the quiz on my website: www.danahmor.com

Vata

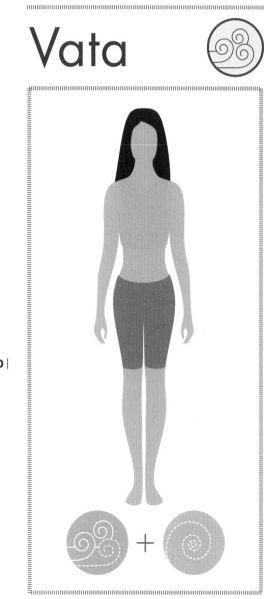

ELEMENT: air, space.
SEASON: winter.
BODY TYPE: thin, delicate bone structure, slender build, low body fat, difficulty gaining weight.
CHARACTERISTICS: sensitive, running late, can't sit still, irregular, forgets to eat, spiritual, routine of the day feels difficult and overwhelming, flightiness, easily confused, enthusiastic, light-headed, creative.

SIGNS OF BALANCE: sharp, quick thinking, creative, fast-talking, abstract.

SIGNS OF IMBALANCE: flatulence, bloating, erratic, unfocused, spacey, dry skin, hair and nails, coldness and chills, nervousness, insomnia, worry, cavities, not too present, memory problems, baldness, dry or rough skin, insomnia, constipation, fatigue, headaches, intolerance to cold, underweight or losing weight, anxiety, worry and restlessness, ADHD.

ORGANS TO NOURISH: nervous system, colon and bones.

FOODS TO REDUCE: low-fat diets, too much raw and cold food, needs careful planning if raw foodie to stay grounded and focused.

FOODS TO INCREASE: warming, lubricating, grounding, heavier foods to calm down, good-quality oils, warming foods and spices to counteract coldness like cinnamon, cayenne and ginger.

BENEFICIAL: warming soups and homemade meals, mashed sweet potatoes, root vegetables, heavier grains, regular meals, routine, weightlifting, Pilates and yoga.

Pitta

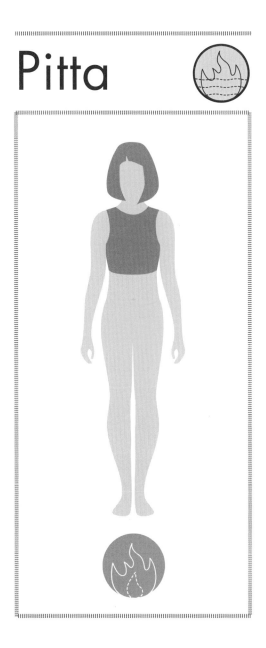

ELEMENT: fire (with a little water)
SEASON: summer.
BODY TYPE: medium body frame, well-proportioned, prone toward muscularity, easily overheated.
CHARACTERISTICS: type A personality, compelled to accomplish things, focused, organized, never misses meals and can be moody if a meal is skipped, workaholic, doesn't do well in hot, humid climates, flirtatious, intelligent, sharp, focused, passionate, entrepreneurial.

SIGNS OF BALANCE: productive, get-it-done person, organized, has a capacity to work until they drop, energized, enthusiastic.

SIGNS OF IMBALANCE: fear, worry, anxiety, skin rashes, inflammatory skin conditions, stomach aches, diarrhoea, controlling and manipulative behaviour, visual problems, excessive body heat, hostility, irritability, excessive competitive drive, easily agitated under stress, angry, irritable, increased appetite, perspiration, over-working.

ORGANS TO NOURISH: liver, gallbladder, spleen, small intestine, blood, eyes.

FOODS TO REDUCE: excessive spices that are too heating, sour foods (lemon is fine), red meat.

FOODS TO INCREASE: bitter and sweet (not sugary) foods (sweet potato, carrots), cooling and astringent, sweet-tasting spices (cardamom, fennel), fresh salads.

BENEFICIAL: fresh mint tea, fresh lime, lighter proteins, dark leafy greens, sweet vegetables, calming and relaxing physical exercise (yoga, Pilates and hiking in nature), gentle relationships.

Kapha

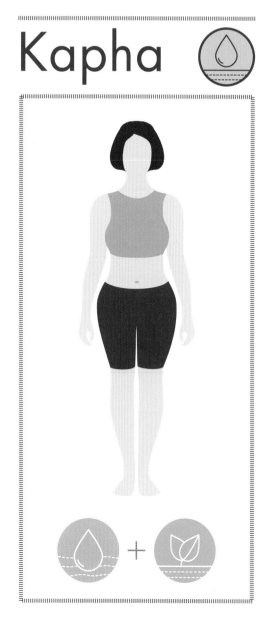

CHARACTERISTICS: easy-going, caring, patient, grounded, stable, solid, sensual, strong libido, sense of physicality, steady appetite (not as strong as pitta), can miss a meal, slower metabolism, resists exercise and is slower moving, often trying to lighten up, can work on for many hours without interruption, strong endurance and stamina.

SIGNS OF BALANCE: reliable, calm, affectionate, caring, loving, peacekeeper, even-tempered.

SIGNS OF IMBALANCE: resistant, possessive, emotional, needy, lethargic, sleeping too much, depressed, lack of enthusiasm, apathetic, feeling dull and sluggish, congestion, overweight, slow digestion, oily skin, sinus congestion, nasal allergies, asthma.

ORGANS TO NOURISH: lungs and respiratory system, stomach, body fat and lymphatic system.

FOODS TO REDUCE: fatty foods, heavy proteins, dairy, gluten, red meats, starchy vegetables.

FOODS TO INCREASE: light grains, light proteins, abundant vegetables, drying and heating foods, heating and pungent spices with thermogenic properties.

BENEFICIAL: sprouted beans, quinoa, spinach, dandelion, salads, cayenne, pepper, ginger, self-acceptance and body-image affirmations, cardiovascular exercises, love the body you have.

ELEMENT: earth and water
SEASON: spring
BODY TYPE: larger body type, gains weight easily (not necessarily overweight), holds fat and water, strong, a powerful athlete when in shape.

GET PRACTICAL – HOW TO APPLY THIS KNOWLEDGE

UNDERSTANDING YOUR BODY AND MOOD

Learn how to understand your own body and mood through the doshas, in relationship to your external environment, food and lifestyle.

The elements in foods will naturally come to you as you grow more conscious and re-establish your relationship with your body and food.

Rather than only focusing on your dosha, it's important to be aware of the current external climate. Your dosha will simply predispose you to the build-up of that element in your body.

For example, a kapha person needs to be more careful in the cold, rainy season. A vata person needs to take more care to stay balanced in the dry, cold winters. Pitta people need to make an extra effort to cool their body down in hot summer weather.

In general, we can all approach each season similarly, living in harmony with nature, eating local and seasonal foods. Nevertheless, in the same season, people with different constitutions may feel very different. In summer for example, a kapha person will feel lighter and healthier, when heat and dryness naturally balances their inner environment they will have less discomfort, less mucus and feel calmer in general. In the same season, a pitta person, being predominantly fire, will have to take care not to overheat and get irritable. Many pitta people ease through the winter months as they feel more relaxed and less fiery, in comparison to those who are predominantly vata or kapha dosha.

HARMONIZE WITH NATURE

DIET & LIFESTYLE FOR THE SEASONS/ DOSHAS & SIMILAR CLIMATES

In Ayurvedic medicine, prevention starts with a lifestyle that is in harmony with the changing cycles of nature.

Eat with the seasons, keep it local, like nature's perfect design – and you will find that you are living in balance with the doshas! The tips on the following pages are most beneficial for each season. However, they can also be applied to you throughout the year to balance your predominant dosha.

For example, those with predominant vata dosha should follow this regimen all year round, and take extra care in the winter months when the elements outside can cause the similar internal element to become aggravated, leading to imbalance.

For example, pitta-dominant people should eat more pitta-pacifying foods all year round, but more importantly in the summer as there is increased fire in the weather and this could cause overheating of the body, resulting in imbalanced emotions and physiology. However, during winter, those of a pitta dosha will find it much easier to keep their overheating predisposition in check because the cooling weather helps them stay cool. They might even find that a spicy dish warms them up and feels good.

We need to follow a regimen devoted to keeping our own elements in balance all year round and take extra care when the season arrives that may aggravate our internal environments.

Knowing your specific dosha is useful because you can gain insight into potential acute situations, discomforts or predispositions to certain conditions – irritability, mucus build-up, congestion, etc. However, nowadays with more people travelling, everchanging climate and non-seasonal foods, it can be easier to go by the season.

GENERAL AYURVEDIC EXERCISE TIPS

VATA: needs calming, light exercise that also soothes your mind. Resistance training and weight lifting also help you stay grounded and strengthen your bones; as you tend to be a thinner build, this is important for bone health.

PITTA: needs moderate amounts of exercise. Long walks in nature, swimming or skiing, which require endurance while the fresh air and nature relax you. In the summer season, pitta dosha should watch out not to overheat, nor over-exercise in the sun.

KAPHA: needs more intense aerobic and stimulating forms of movement. Try a cross trainer (elyptical), as it causes less impact and protects your joints. Sweating and sauna are perfect ways to complete your movement sessions.

Autumn, winter and spring are the perfect seasons to embrace more stimulating movement. During the summer, avoid overheating and working out in the hot sun.

BENEFITS OF AYURVEDA

Nutrition can be confusing. It is the only science where there are numerous contradictory claims. With the ever-changing hi-tech industry and new discoveries, even doctors are concerned about how an average child or adult in any country can understand what is beneficial for him/her when doctors are not entirely sure about diet advice themselves.

Ayurveda invites us to understand our own bodies so that we can excel as unique beings, and make the best food and lifestyle choices for ourselves and in the different seasons. We cannot be grouped by gender for calorie intake, by blood group, or by age, because we are all different and our bodies are constantly changing their internal environments. What may be beneficial for you on a sunny day may be harmful for you in the winter. By understanding the elements that make up our body and mind we can understand ourselves better and actually improve our inner communication thanks to the ancient wisdom of Ayurveda.

VATA/WINTER

Vata dosha and winter tips that are the most nourishing during the cooler and dryer vata months of winter.

EAT MORE
Salty/heavy, sour, sweet (not sugary), oily (tahini and almond), moist, warm: soups, stews, curries, steamed veggies, grains, herbal teas, dark green leaves in the winter will boost immunity, add warming foods like onions, and a rich and warming salad dressing.

EAT LESS
Spicy, bitter, astringent/light, cold as they dry and cool the body.

PACIFYING HERBS (TO BALANCE AND REDUCE EXCESS VATA)
Anise, asafoetida, black pepper, cinnamon, coriander, clove, cumin, fennel, garlic, ginger, mustard seeds.

VATA/WINTER ROUTINES:
* Add ghee, avocado, sesame or olive oil to your grains and soups
* Follow a regular rhythm of sleep, exercise, mealtimes and rest
* Self-massage with warm raw sesame oil in a warming bath.

SIGNS OF EXCESS VATA:
Insomnia, stress, worry, constipation, colds and flus, joint pain.

PITTA/SUMMER

Pitta dosha and summer tips that are the most nourishing during the hot and dry pitta months of summer.

EAT MORE
Sweet, bitter, astringent, fresh foods such as salads, leafy greens, smoothies, fresh seasonal fruit.

EAT LESS
Pungent (spicy), sour, salty, dry spicy foods, alcohol.

PACIFYING HERBS (TO BALANCE AND REDUCE EXCESS PITTA)
Cardamom, fennel, fresh mint, coriander seeds, chicory, dandelion.

PITTA/SUMMER ROUTINES
* Walking in green nature
* Swimming – things that keep you cool, fresh and calm
* Drink a lot of water
* Self-massage with coconut oil
* Avoid excessive activity during midday heat as it can be draining

SIGNS OF EXCESS PITTA:
Irritability and impatience, heartburn, acid reflux, stomach ulcers, sensitivity to heat, lethargy, sarcasm, skin rashes, boils, acne, low blood sugar, difficulty falling asleep.

KAPHA/SPRING

Stay strong and healthy during spring and cold, rainy weather.

EAT MORE
Pungent (spicy), bitter, astringent/light, dry, warm foods: mostly plant based is best such as flavourful steamed veggies, broth soups, quinoa, millet and buckwheat, sprouts and seeds (chia, sesame and sunflower seeds).

EAT LESS
Sweet, sour, salty/heavy, cold, oily: such as fried/oily foods/drinks, ice cream, heavy dairy, animal protein, cold iced drinks, wheat and couscous, sweet fruits like bananas and mangos or heavy nuts like brazil nuts and macadamia nuts.

PACIFYING HERBS (TO BALANCE AND REDUCE EXCESS KAPHA)
Anise, asafoetida, cayenne (uncooked), cinnamon, clove, mustard seed, basil, bay leaf, black pepper, chamomile, caraway, cardamom, coriander, dill, fennel, fenugreek, garlic, ginger, horseradish, marjoram, nutmeg, oregano, peppermint, poppy seeds, rosemary, saffron, sage, spearmint, thyme, turmeric.

KAPHA/SPRING ROUTINES
* *Stimulating movement like brisk walking in the morning to increase circulation, mood, and immunity*
* *Self-massage with warm raw sesame oil*
* *Neti – irrigating your nasal passage with warm salt water (always follow with nasya)*
* *Nasya – dip a q-tip in warm sesame oil, swirl it inside your nostrils, and inhale deeply*
* *Yoga postures that are stimulating and energizing like sun salutations and cat pose*
* *Eat only when hungry. Allow the body time for digestion*

SIGNS OF EXCESS KAPHA:
Cold, cough, allergies, congestion, flu, fatigue, depression, weight gain.

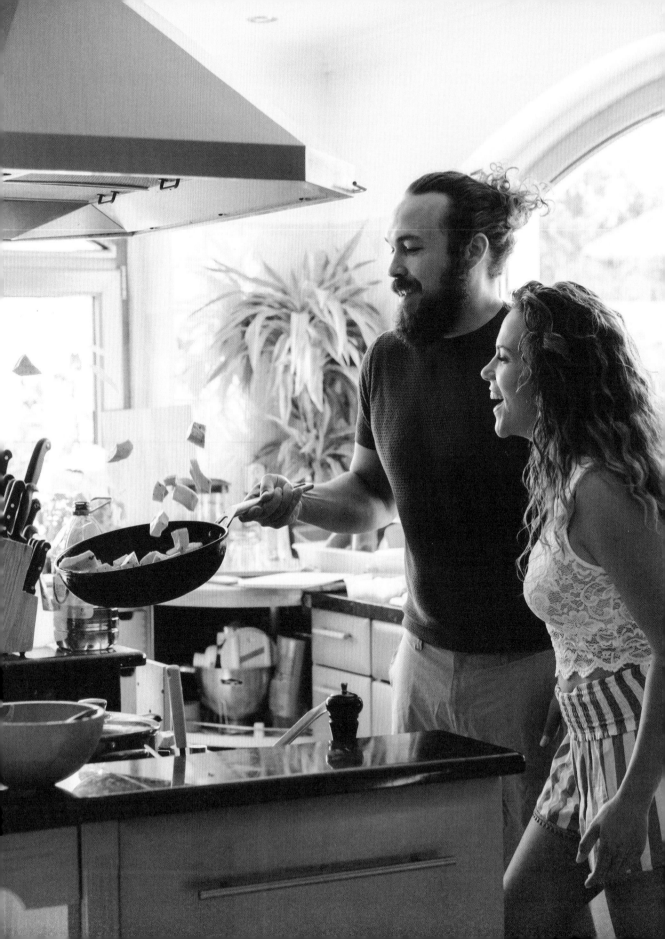

MEAL PLANNING & TIPS

When trying to implement changes in your relationship with food, it can sometimes be hard to look at the week and visualize what you are going to eat to stay on course. With that in mind, I've written this section to supply you with inspiration and give you vision. Below are a few meal plan ideas to get you started on your journey.

BREAKING-THE-FAST

Now that you have worked through the book and know that breaking-the-fast is about prolonging toxic elimination, here are a few good ideas that allow the body to continue its daily detox, rehydrate after the night and fill you with nutrients first thing in the morning.

* *Lemon water*
* *Green juice (p.187)*
* *Mean Green Smoothie (p.187).*

MORNING SNACK

If you're really hungry or your morning is super active and you can't last till lunch, having a nutritious mid-morning snack to hand is a great way of avoiding falling back on sugar-loaded convenience foods. Try something from my Sexy Snacks list on page 271.

LUNCH AND DINNER

For me, lunch is always the largest and most nutritious meal of the day as this is when your body is fully awake and its digestive powers are at their highest.

Dinner is best eaten as a lighter meal than lunch. This helps with digestion and prepares your body for sleep – which is when the body begins its daily detox. The earlier and lighter your dinner is, the better your nighttime recovery will be.

How to make a smashing salad

In the warmer months my lunch is usually a huge salad topped with all kinds of exciting extras – these can be anything from nuts and seeds to roasted veggies leftover from the previous evening's meal. To keep your salads varied, flavoursome and exciting it's important to vary the ingredients that you use.

Yummy extras to add to your salad:
*   sautéed asparagus
*   steamed veggies
*   sautéed veggies with garlic
*   endives (chopped and marinated with lemon juice and olive oil, or boiled)
*   roasted sweet potato
*   grilled (broiled) or roasted veggies
*   boiled potatoes/sweet potatoes, pumpkin and steamed green beans
*   tahini
*   hummus
*   sauerkraut and other fermented foods
*   sprouts (clover, mung beans, fenugreek seeds, sprouted lentils, etc.)
*   purple cabbage with lemon juice, olive oil and garlic
*   roasted (bell) peppers in olive oil
*   mixed seeds
*   balsamic glaze

The other thing that I always have ready and waiting in the fridge is a delicious dressing! Use lemon and olive oil as a base for your dressings and be creative from there. Adding pesto, tahini, tamari or umeboshi plum vinegar, or herbs and spices such as paprika will spice it up and make it delicious! For a creamy dressing, I sometimes add a little coconut yogurt.

Meal ideas

For inspiration, some of my favourite meals are listed below:
*   barbecue-style portobello mushrooms with quinoa pilaf
*   dhal with brown basmati rice and fresh coriander (cilantro) chutney
*   courgette (zucchini) spaghetti with fresh pesto and sautéed tomatoes
*   black bean stew with quinoa
*   oven roasted veggies served with millet purée and salad
*   baked tomato and chickpea curry
*   baked stuffed courgettes (zucchini)
*   pumpkin risotto (wholegrain rice)
*   veggie burgers with sweet potato chips and tahini dip
*   risotto al fungi (wholegrain rice) with basil pesto
*   veggie pie with a crunchy base (made with chickpea flour), served with salad and balsamic glaze

MY FAVOURITE SEXY SNACKS

* overnight oats
* energizing granola bowl
* buckwheat pancakes and avocado
* hummus with raw veggies (carrots, cucumbers, endives, sliced peppers)
* tahini with cucumbers (my favourite lazy dinner!)
* mashed avocado or guacamole with rice crackers or oven-baked tortilla chips
* sweet potato wedges with tahini, hummus or pesto
* gluten-free toast or rice crackers with avocado slices
* gluten-free pancakes with sunflower spread and tomato slices
* almond trail mix
* lightly salted popcorn with spices (cumin and pepper work well)
* artichoke with lemon, garlic and olive oil dip
* Danah Banana's Smoothie: frozen banana, almond butter, chia seeds, almond milk, spirulina powder and cacao powder blended until smooth.

BON COURAGE!

Whatever you takeaway from this book – whether it's ditching dairy or gluten or starting a dance class – remember that these steps are creating new habits and neural pathways. Whatever you decide to do, keep it fun! That way you're more likely to want to do it again tomorrow!

Remember that there are two forms of food: secondary foods that only nourish the body, while primary foods have the capacity to feed your spirit and nourish your being far beyond any physical food. Don't confuse the two!

Be brave, be yourself! Often, we carry an image of ourselves that has been projected onto us by others, but having the courage to be yourself can set you free.

Thank you for being part of this journey with me and having the willingness to open and read this book! I hope it brings you health, vitality and sunshine!

Danah

ACKNOWLEDGEMENTS

When I graduated high school I took a journey that was a little different from most of my friends. On this journey I met many incredible people, teachers, professors and doctors from all corners of the world, all of whom left their mark on me in a special way. I want to thank each of them for opening their worlds and sharing their passion, wisdom and knowledge with me.

Writing a book can be very isolating and I want to thank all my friends and family who made this experience less solitary and who were always there to debrief over a very late dinner or at the end of the phone to ask how things were going. Thank you for your love and support!

Thank you to everyone who is reading this book. You were, and continue to be my main motivation.

To Catarina, who was there from the very start of this project supporting my crazy ideas and encouraging me in every way. I thank you!

To Pat, who believed in me and motivated my writing. I know you're looking down on me and you're proud. Mazal tov.

Thank you to Amanda, who calmed me down when I got stressed and made me feel it was OK to communicate my truth. Thank you to Fred for believing in this project!

To Sophie, my dear copy editor – it has been such a pleasure to work with you! I can't thank you enough for your dedication and wonderful personality!

To Jo, Dan and Fra at Watkins, it has been such a great experience to work with you and a pleasure to get to know you! I'm looking forward to working together on future projects. Thank you for believing in MorLife!

To Mum and Dad, I couldn't feel more grateful to have you as my parents and guides to the world. Thank you for educating me with an open mind, supporting my crazy dreams and for always encouraging me to stand up for what I believe in. Mum – you have always expected nothing less than my best, and I thank you for showing me this way of life! You are an inspiring woman. Thank you for seeing me and being a friend.

To my brother, Nathanael and sister, Maya – you guys are my soulmates. Thank you for all the fun we have together, for being a part of this project. Nati, my buddy-in-crime in the kitchen, thanks for your delicious food and flavours! I can't wait to get the cookbook out! Maya, for your creative inspiration and illustrations. I love you both!